the**clinics.com**

CLINICS IN FAMILY PRACTICE

Rheumatology

GUEST EDITOR
James M. Gill, MD, MPH

CONSULTING EDITOR
Barbara S. Apgar, MD, MS

June 2005 • Volume 7 • Number 2

SAUNDERS

An Imprint of Elsevier, Inc.
PHILADELPHIA   LONDON   TORONTO   MONTREAL   SYDNEY   TOKYO

W.B. SAUNDERS COMPANY
A Division of Elsevier Inc.

1600 John F. Kennedy Boulevard • Suite 1800 • Philadelphia, Pennsylvania 19103
http://www.theclinics.com

CLINICS IN FAMILY PRACTICE   Volume 7, Number 2
June 2005   ISSN 1522-5720
Editor: J. Heather Cullen   ISBN 1-4160-2659-2

The ideas and opinions expressed in *Clinics in Family Practice* do not necessarily reflect those of the Publisher. The Publisher does not assume any responsibility of any injury and/or damage to persons or property arising out of or related to any use of the material contained in this periodical. The reader is advised to check the appropriate medical literature and the product information currently provided by the manufacturer of each drug to be administered to verify the dosage, the method and duration of administration, or contraindications. It is the responsibility of the treating physician or other health care professional, relying on independent experience and knowledge of the patient, to determine drug dosages and the best treatment for the patient. Mention of any product in this issue should not be construed as endorsement by the contributors, editors, or the Publisher of the product or manufacturers' claims.

Clinics in Family Practice (ISSN 1522-5720) is published quarterly by W.B. Saunders Company, 360 Park Avenue South, New York, NY 10010. Corporate and Editorial Offices: 170 S. Independence Mall W, Suite 300E, Philadelphia, PA 19106-3399. Subscription prices are $115.00 per year (US individuals), $159.00 per year (US institutions), $58.00 per year (US students), $132.00 per year (Canadian individuals), $192.00 per year (Canadian institutions), $132.00 per year (Canadian individuals), $145.00 per year (foreign individuals), $192.00 per year (foreign institutions), and $73.00 per year (foreign students). Foreign air speed delivery is included in all *Clinics* subscription prices. All prices are subject to change without notice. Customer Service: 1-800-654-2452. (US). From outside of the US, call 1-407-345-4000. E-mail: hhspcs@harcourt.com.

Application to mail at Periodicals postage rate is pending at New York, NY and additional offices.

POSTMASTER: Send address changes to *Clinics in Family Practice*, W.B. Saunders Company, Periodicals Customer Service, Orlando, FL 32887-4800.

Printed in the United States of America.

CONSULTING EDITOR

BARBARA S. APGAR, MD, MS, Clinical Professor of Family Medicine, University of Michigan Medical School, Chelsea, Michigan

GUEST EDITOR

JAMES M. GILL, MD, MPH, Associate Professor, Department of Family Medicine; Senior Scientist, Department of Health Policy, Jefferson Medical College, Philadelphia, Pennsylvania; Director, Department of Family and Community Medicine, Health Services Research, Christiana Care Health Services, Wilmington, Delaware

CONTRIBUTORS

PETER J. CAREK, MD, MS, Director, Trident/MUSC Family Medicine Residency Program, Medical University of South Carolina; and Associate Professor of Family Medicine, Department of Family Medicine, Medical University of South Carolina, Charleston, South Carolina

RAJWINDER S. DEU, MD, Primary Care Sports Medicine Fellow, Department of Family Medicine, Thomas Jefferson University, Philadelphia, Pennsylvania

JOHN A. DONNELLY, MD, Faculty, Department of Internal Medicine and Pediatrics, Christiana Care Health Systems, Newark, Delaware

HEATHER BITTNER FAGAN, MD, Director of Faculty Development Program, Assistant Director of Health Services Research, Department of Family and Community Medicine, Christiana Care Health System, Wilmington, Delaware; and Assistant Professor, Department of Family Medicine, Thomas Jefferson University, Philadelphia, Pennsylvania

ANDREW J. FOY, Jr, BS, Jefferson Medical College, Philadelphia, Pennsylvania

JAMES M. GILL, MD, MPH, Associate Professor, Department of Family Medicine; Senior Scientist, Department of Health Policy, Jefferson Medical College, Philadelphia, Pennsylvania; Director, Department of Family and Community Medicine, Health Services Research, Christiana Care Health Services, Wilmington, Delaware

GINA GILL GLASS, MD, Olde Towne Medical Center, Williamsburg, Virginia

MARC I. HARWOOD, MD, Assistant Professor; Assistant Residency Director, Department of Family Medicine; and Assistant Director, Sports Medicine Fellowship Program, Jefferson Medical College, Thomas Jefferson University, Philadelphia, Pennsylvania

MELISSA H. HUNTER, MD, Associate Professor, Department of Family Medicine, Medical University of South Carolina, Charleston, South Carolina

ESHWAR KAPUR, MD, Fellow, Primary Care Sports Medicine, Department of Family Medicine, Jefferson Medical College, Thomas Jefferson University, Philadelphia, Pennsylvania

JOHN R. LAWRENCE, MD, Department of Family and Community Medicine, Christiana Care Health Services, Wilmington, Delaware

JENNIFER NATICCHIA, MD, Clinical Instructor, Department of Family Medicine, Jefferson Medical College, Thomas Jefferson University Hospital, Philadelphia, Pennsylvania; Residency Director, Department of Family and Community Medicine, Christiana Care Health System, Wilmington, Delaware

JANICE E. NEVIN, MD, MPH, Chair, Department of Family and Community Medicine, Christiana Care Health System, Wilmington, Delaware; Associate Professor of Family Medicine, Jefferson Medical College, Philadelphia, Pennsylvania

JAMES H. NEWMAN, MD, FACP, Associate Chief Medical Officer and Chief, Section of Rheumatology, Christiana Care Health System, Wilmington, Delaware

ANNA QUISEL, MD, Private Practice, Wilmington, Delaware

BROOKE E. SALZMAN, MD, Fellow in Geriatrics, Department of Family Medicine, Thomas Jefferson University Hospital, Philadelphia, Pennsylvania

BRADLEY J. SMITH, MD, Resident, Family Medicine Residency Program, Department of Family Medicine, Jefferson Medical College, Thomas Jefferson University, Philadelphia, Pennsylvania

JAMES STUDDIFORD, MD, FACP, Jefferson Medical College, Philadelphia, Pennsylvania

MARCIA L. TAYLOR, MD, Instructor, Department of Family Medicine, Medical University of South Carolina, Charleston, South Carolina

SETH TORREGIANI, DO, Resident, Department of Internal Medicine and Pediatrics, Christiana Care Health Systems, Newark, Delaware

DYANNE P. WESTERBERG, DO, Department of Family and Community Medicine, Christiana Care Health Services, Wilmington, Delaware

CONTENTS

Low Back Pain: A Primary Care Approach 279

Marc I. Harwood and Bradley J. Smith

Low back pain (LBP) is a common presenting complaint in the primary care setting. Most patients with LBP have spontaneous resolution of their symptoms. It is important to be able to quickly differentiate the more serious causes of LBP from the self-limited etiologies. This article discusses diagnostic considerations, including physical examination and imaging findings, and management options for patients with LBP.

Approach to the Patient with Acute Swollen/Painful Joint 305

Heather Bittner Fagan

The approach to the patient with the acutely painful or swollen joint is determined by history and physical examination. First, the clinician must distinguish arthralgia from arthritis. Next, the clinician must consider the location, the number of joints involved, localization (articular versus nonarticular), duration, and associated symptoms. The approach to the patient with monoarticular joint pain varies significantly from the approach to the patient with polyarticular joint pain. In this article we focus on pain or swelling in a single joint (monarthritis) or a small number of joints (oligoarthritis). The acute, swollen painful joint or acute monoarthritis is a potential medical emergency, and prompt attention is needed to provide appropriate therapy in a timely manner. History, physical examination, and synovial fluid testing are the key tools in diagnosis.

Approach to the Patient with Raynaud's Phenomenon 321

Dyanne P. Westerberg and John R. Lawrence

Raynaud's phenomenon is a condition of episodic, reversible, vasospastic digital ischemia. It manifests classically as the sequential development of a three-phase color change of blanching, cyanosis, and rubor after cold exposure and subsequent rewarming. This article discusses the background, diagnosis, and treatment of Raynaud's phenomenon.

A Primary Care Approach to the Use and Interpretation of Common Rheumatologic Tests 335

Brooke E. Salzman, Janice E. Nevin, and James H. Newman

The results of common rheumatologic laboratory tests play an important part in the diagnosis and management of rheumatic diseases. This article describes the characteristics of commonly ordered rheumatologic tests and reviews examples of their application in a primary care setting.

In 1951, Hollander introduced local corticosteroid injection therapy for the treatment of inflammatory arthritis. Since that time, aspiration of synovial fluid and injection of joints, bursae, tendon sheaths, and soft tissues are frequently used diagnostic and therapeutic skills for many physicians practicing in the outpatient setting. This article discusses joint and soft tissue injections in the primary care setting.

FORTHCOMING ISSUES

RECENT ISSUES

PREFACE

"Doctor, my knees hurt." "Doctor, my muscles hurt." Musculoskeletal pain is one of the most common complaints that is encountered in office practice [1]. In 2002, musculoskeletal and connective tissue problems accounted for more than 66 million office visits. Nonsteroidal anti-inflammatory drugs (NSAIDs), which often are used for musculoskeletal pain, were the most common class of medication prescribed or recommended during office visits [1].

Musculoskeletal pain can be particularly challenging for primary care clinicians because patients usually present with nonspecific problems. For example, arthropathies are one of the most common categories of illnesses seen by primary care clinicians [1]; however, when a patient presents with acute joint pain and swelling, the differential diagnosis is wide and varied. The problem may be self-limited, such as temporary swelling that is due to a minor injury. It may be an exacerbation of a chronic disease, such as osteoarthritis. Or it can be an illness that is threatening to life or limb, such as lupus or a septic joint.

Interpretation of rheumatologic laboratory tests also can be daunting. Who among our primary care colleagues has not been uncertain about the significance of a positive antinuclear antibody (ANA) test? Causing more uncertainty is deciding the next test to order. Is it appropriate to order additional rheumatologic tests to rule in or rule out a serious disease, such as lupus? If so, is it best to order specific auto-antibody tests, or is there a general "lupus panel"? Or is the best course of action to refer to a rheumatologist?

Medication choices also can be confusing. Even for common and straightforward conditions, such as osteoarthritis, the choice of medications is growing. For pain control, does acetaminophen work just as well as NSAIDs? What about Cox-2 inhibitors? Initially, it was believed that they would simplify management of musculoskeletal pain, because they were believed to be safer and more effective than traditional NSAIDs; however, there is now evidence of increased cardiovascular risk with Cox-2 inhibitors. So weighing the risks and benefits may have become even more complicated.

The purpose of this issue of *Clinics of Family Practice* is to assist primary care clinicians in addressing these difficult issues in the common but often confusing field of rheumatology. Each article addresses a topic related to rheumatology or the management of musculoskeletal problems. We have included the most common rheumatologic conditions that are encountered by primary care clinicians, such as osteoarthritis and fibromyalgia. Also included are rheumatologic conditions that are less common but potentially serious, such as Lyme disease, systemic lupus erythematosus, polymyalgia rheumatica, and giant cell arteritis.

We also have included several articles on common musculoskeletal and sports injuries. Such common upper extremity injuries, such as trigger finger and carpal tunnel syndrome, are addressed. We have also included underrecognized injuries of the hip and groin, such as sportsman's hernia and osteitis pubis. Although these conditions usually are not considered in the medical specialty of rheumatology, they are included in the differential diagnosis of musculoskeletal pain. In the primary care setting, symptoms often are vague and problems often are not yet diagnosed, so the distinction between medical rheumatology and musculoskeletal injury often is unclear.

Because primary care clinicians often encounter problems that are undiagnosed, we also have included articles that are problem-oriented rather than disease-oriented. The articles on back pain, acute joint pain, and Raynaud's syndrome are designed to help clinicians approach problems that are undifferentiated, and that may or may not be due to an underlying diagnosis. The article on abnormal rheumatologic labs is designed to help the primary care clinician sort through the conundrum of what to do with an abnormal ANA or an abnormal erythrocyte sedimentation rate. Finally, we have included an article to assist primary care clinicians with the most common office-based procedures in musculoskeletal medicine: joint aspiration and injection.

Each of these articles is written for the particular needs of the primary care clinician. Each includes key points, tables, and other summaries to make the recommendations easy to use. Just as important, each article uses an evidence-based approach. The recommendations are based upon the best available evidence, and each major recommendation is given a grade to reflect the strength of that evidence.

EVIDENCE-BASED MEDICINE IN PRIMARY CARE

First, it is important to understand what evidence-based medicine (EBM) is. Simply stated, EBM is the "conscientious, explicit and judicious use of current best evidence in making decisions about the care of individual patients" [2]. An evidence-based approach requires that physicians ask themselves a specific question whenever a test or treatment is considered: "Is there evidence that this test (or treatment) provides more benefit than risk?". An evidence-based approach does not require that physicians ignore the importance of clinical experience. Rather, it requires that physicians combine clinical experience with the best scientific evidence to make their decisions.

It may seem obvious that we would want to treat our patients based on the best scientific evidence in combination with good clinical judgment; however, practicing EBM is not always easy. It is impractical for busy practicing clinicians to review and summarize the primary literature each time that they have a clinical question. Therefore, we usually rely on clinical reviews that summarize the literature and make recommendations based on these summaries. Although these clinical reviews often are easy to use, they often are not based on the best available evidence. The most valuable information sources for practicing physicians are those that are easy to use and evidence-based. That is the goal of the articles in this issue of *Clinics of Family Practice*: to provide an easy-to-use evidence-based review for a variety of topics in the field of rheumatology.

This evidence-based approach to clinical reviews is not a new concept. Many of the major sources of information for primary care physicians have moved to an evidence-based format. For example, the *Journal of Family Practice* and *American Family Physician* now require reviews to be evidence-based. All of the recommendations in these journals are graded on the quality of the evidence. This issue of *Clinics in Family Practice* follows a similar evidence-based approach, and uses the same evidence grading system that is used in the *Journal of Family Practice*.

EVIDENCE-BASED GRADING SYSTEM

Readers need to understand the strength of the evidence on which a clinical review recommendation is based before deciding whether to follow that recommendation. In cancer screening, for example, there is strong evidence that mammograms benefit women ages 50 to 69. So it would be difficult for family physicians to ignore the strong recommendation to order mammograms for women in this age group. Conversely, the evidence for the benefit of prostate cancer screening is weak, and organizations that follow an evidence-based approach generally do not recommend routine screening. Rather, they recommend that the decision be based on a discussion of the risks and benefits and a mutual decision between the physician and patient. Physicians have much more flexibility in deciding whether to recommend prostate cancer screening and in presenting it to patients.

To reflect the quality of evidence and strength of recommendation in our articles, we used the "Oxford Centre for Evidence-based Medicine Levels of Evidence." As with most evidence-grading systems, this system uses two steps. First, the quality of the evidence is assessed. For studies of treatment, high-quality randomized clinical trials (RCTs) and systematic reviews of RCTs are assigned the highest level of evidence (level 1), followed respectively by cohort studies, case-control studies, case series, and expert opinion (which is given the lowest level of evidence, at level 5). In the second step, the strength of recommendation is graded based on the level of evidence. Recommendations that are based on the highest level of evidence (level 1) are given the highest grade (Grade A). Recommendations that are based on expert opinion only (level 5) are given the lowest grade (Grade D). A more detailed description of the grading system for evidence and recommendations is shown in the Appendix.

Although it is important that information sources for primary care clinicians be evidence based, it also is important that they be easy to use. It can be frustrating to a busy practicing physician to have to read through an entire article to glean the key information that is needed to make clinical decisions. Therefore, the articles in this issue also have brief summaries of key points, and tables that summarize the major recommendations. These summaries include the grades of the recommendations, so that clinicians can know the strength of evidence upon which the recommendations are based. Through providing a series of articles on common conditions, with recommendations that are evidence-based and easy to use, we hope to help practicing primary care clinicians to be more confident in the difficult and often confusing field of rheumatology and musculoskeletal pain.

JAMES M. GILL, MD, MPH
Guest Editor
Christiana Care Health Services
Department of Family and Community Medicine
1401 Foulk Road
Wilmington, DE 19803, USA
E-mail: jgill@christianacare.org

References

[1] Woodwell DA, Cherry DK. *2002* Summary: National Ambulatory Medical Care Survey. Hyattsville (MD): Advance data from vital and health Statistics; No. 36; 2004.
[2] Geyman JP. Evidence-based medicine in primary care: an overview. J Am Board Fam Pract 1998;11(1):46–56.

APPENDIX

Oxford Centre for Evidence-based Medicine Levels of Evidence (May 2001)

Level	Therapy/ Prevention, Etiology/Harm	Prognosis	Diagnosis	Differential Diagnosis/Symptom Prevalence Study	Economic and Decision Analyses
1a	SR (with homogeneity*) of RCTs	SR (with homogeneity*) of inception cohort studies; CDR[†] validated in different populations	SR (with homogeneity*) of Level 1 diagnostic studies; CDR[†] with 1b studies from different clinical centers	SR (with homogeneity*) of prospective cohort studies	SR (with homogeneity*) of Level 1 economic studies
1b	Individual RCT (with narrow confidence interval[‡])	Individual inception cohort study with ≥80% follow-up; CDR[†] validated in a single population	Validating** cohort study with good[†††] reference standards; or CDR[†] tested within one clinical center	Prospective cohort study with good follow-up[****]	Analysis based on clinically sensible costs or alternatives; systematic review(s) of the evidence; and including multi-way sensitivity analyses
1c	All or none[§]	All or none case-series	Absolute SpPins and SnNouts[††]	All or none case-series	Absolute better-value[‡‡] or worse-value analyses[††††]
2a	SR (with homogeneity*) of cohort studies	SR (with homogeneity*) of either retrospective cohort studies or untreated control groups in RCTs	SR (with homogeneity*) of Level >2 diagnostic studies	SR (with homogeneity*) of 2b and better studies	SR (with homogeneity*) of Level >2 economic studies

(continued on next page)

Level	Therapy/Prevention, Etiology/Harm	Prognosis	Diagnosis	Differential Diagnosis/Symptom Prevalence Study	Economic and Decision Analyses
2b	Individual cohort study (including low quality RCT; eg, <80% follow-up)	Retrospective cohort study or follow-up of untreated control patients in an RCT; Derivation of CDR† or validated on split-sample§§§ only	Exploratory** cohort study with good††reference standards; CDR† after derivation, or validated only on split-sample§§§ or databases	Retrospective cohort study, or poor follow-up	Analysis based on clinically sensible costs or alternatives; limited review(s) of the evidence, or single studies; and including multi-way sensitivity analyses
2c	"Outcomes" research; Ecological studies	"Outcomes" research		Ecological studies	Audit or outcomes research
3a	SR (with homogeneity*) of case-control studies		SR (with homogeneity*) of 3b and better studies	SR (with homogeneity*) of 3b and better studies	SR (with homogeneity*) of 3b and better studies
3b	Individual case-control study		Nonconsecutive study; or without consistently applied reference standards	Nonconsecutive cohort study, or very limited population	Analysis based on limited alternatives or costs, poor quality estimates of data, but including sensitivity analyses incorporating clinically sensible variations.
4	Case-series (and poor quality cohort and case-control studies§§)	Case-series (and poor quality prognostic cohort studies***)	Case-control study, poor or nonindependent reference standard	Case-series or superseded reference standards	Analysis with no sensitivity analysis
5	Expert opinion without explicit critical appraisal, or based on physiology, bench research or "first principles"	Expert opinion without explicit critical appraisal, or based on physiology, bench research or "first principles"	Expert opinion without explicit critical appraisal, or based on physiology, bench research or "first principles"	Expert opinion without explicit critical appraisal, or based on physiology, bench research or "first principles"	Expert opinion without explicit critical appraisal, or based on economic theory or "first principles"

Produced by Bob Phillips, Chris Ball, Dave Sackett, Doug Badenoch, Sharon Straus, Brian Haynes, Martin Dawes since November 1998.

Notes

Users can add a minus-sign "–" to denote the level of that fails to provide a conclusive answer because of:

- EITHER a single result with a wide confidence interval (such that, for example, an ARR in an RCT is not statistically significant but whose confidence intervals fail to exclude clinically important benefit or harm)
- Or a systematic review with troublesome (and statistically significant) heterogeneity.

* Such evidence is inconclusive, and therefore, only can generate Grade D recommendations.

† By homogeneity we mean a systematic review that is free of worrisome variations (heterogeneity) in the directions and degrees of results between individual studies. Not all systematic reviews with statistically significant heterogeneity need be worrisome, and not all worrisome heterogeneity need be statistically significant. As noted above, studies displaying worrisome heterogeneity should be tagged with a "–" at the end of their designated level.

‡ Clinical decision rule. (These are algorithms or scoring systems which lead to a prognostic estimation or a diagnostic category.)

‡ See note #2 for advice on how to understand, rate and use trials or other studies with wide confidence intervals.

§ Met when all patients died before the Rx became available, but some now survive on it; or when some patients died before the Rx became available, but none now die on it.

§§ By poor quality cohort study we mean one that failed to define comparison groups clearly or failed to measure exposures and outcomes in the same (preferably blinded), objective way in exposed and nonexposed individuals or failed to identify or appropriately control known confounders or failed to carry out a sufficiently long and complete follow-up of patients. By poor quality case-control study we mean one that failed to define comparison groups clearly or failed to measure exposures and outcomes in the same (preferably blinded), objective way in cases and controls or failed to identify or appropriately control known confounders.

§§§ Split-sample validation is achieved by collecting all the information in a single tranche, then artificially dividing this into "derivation" and "validation" samples.

†† An "Absolute SpPin" is a diagnostic finding whose Specificity is so high that a Positive result rules-in the diagnosis. An "Absolute SnNout" is a diagnostic finding whose Sensitivity is so high that a Negative result rules-out the diagnosis.

‡‡ Good, better, bad, and worse refer to the comparisons between treatments in terms of their clinical risks and benefits.

††† Good reference standards are independent of the test, and applied blindly or objectively to all patients. Poor reference standards are applied haphazardly, but still independent of the test. Use of a nonindependent reference standard (where the 'test' is included in the 'reference', or where the 'testing' affects the 'reference') implies a level 4 study.

†††† Better-value treatments are clearly as good but less expensive, or better at the same or reduced cost. Worse-value treatments are as good and more expensive, or worse and equally or more expensive.

*** Validating studies test the quality of a specific diagnostic test, based on earlier evidence. An exploratory study collects information and trawls the data (eg, using a regression analysis) to find which factors are 'significant'.

**** By poor quality prognostic cohort study we mean one in which sampling was biased in favor of patients who already had the target outcome, or the measurement of outcomes was accomplished in <80% of study patients, or outcomes were determined in an unblinded, nonobjective way, or there was no correction for confounding factors.

**** Good follow-up in a differential diagnosis study is >80%, with adequate time for alternative diagnoses to emerge (eg, 1–6 months acute, 1–5 years chronic).

Grades of recommendation

A   consistent level 1 studies
B   consistent level 2 or 3 studies or extrapolations from level 1 studies
C   level 4 studies or extrapolations from level 2 or 3 studies
D   level 5 evidence or troublingly inconsistent or inconclusive studies of any level

"Extrapolations" are where data is used in a situation which has potentially clinically important differences than the original study situation. *From* Center for Evidence Based Medicine, Oxford, UK. Available at http://www.cebm.net/levels_of_evidence.asp; with permission.

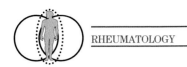
OSTEOARTHRITIS

Gina Gill Glass, MD

Osteoarthritis (OA) is a prevalent rheumatic disease characterized by the progressive breakdown of articular cartilage, resulting in pain, deformity, and decreased function of affected joints. Degenerative joint disease is another term used to describe this condition. Nearly all persons aged 65 to 74 have been shown to have radiographic evidence of OA in their hands. Only 11.2% of these patients report symptoms of hand OA [1].

OA is a major cause of dysfunction and disability. Arthritic disorders are the most common cause of disability in adults [2], and OA is the most prevalent type of arthritis. Risk factors for OA include advanced age, female gender, genetic predisposition, obesity, and joint injury (including trauma, repetitive use, and prior inflammation). OA can develop as a secondary consequence of congenital or developmental joint disorders and of metabolic or endocrine diseases [3,4].

The etiology of OA is unclear. Mechanical, biochemical, and genetic factors seem to play a role. Articular cartilage is primarily composed of extracellular matrix, with chondrocytes comprising only 1% to 2% of its volume. The major components of the extracellular matrix are water, collagen, and proteoglycans. Chondrocytes synthesize the latter two components [4]. One theory is that increased levels of cytokines, such as interleukin-1 and tumor necrosis factor-α, prompt chondrocytes to release enzymes that break down the extracellular matrix. Simultaneously, there is a decrease in the substances that usually inhibit this breakdown. The cartilage breakdown products seem to promote further inflammation, continuing this cycle of cartilage breakdown. Osteophyte formation and other alterations in joint architecture are end results. How or why this cycle starts is uncertain. The data supporting this theory are mainly from animal studies using secondary arthritis as a model. These models have revealed that inflammation may be a more important component of the development and progression of OA than was once thought [3–5].

From the Olde Towne Medical Center, Williamsburg, Virginia

CLINICAL PRESENTATION AND DIAGNOSIS

Typical symptoms of OA include gradual onset of pain and stiffness in and around a joint with decreased function of that joint. Early in the disease process, the pain is typically mild, worsening with use of the affected joint and improving with rest of the joint. If present, morning stiffness rarely lasts more than 30 minutes. Stiffness is common after inactivity of the joint, usually resolving after a few minutes. Pain at rest or at night occurs in more severe disease [6].

Joints affected by OA include knees; hips; cervical and lumbar spine; the first metatarsophalangeal joints of the feet; and distal interphalangeal (DIP), proximal interphalangeal (PIP), and first carpometacarpal (CMC) joints of the hand. Patients with knee OA may complain of "buckling," especially while descending stairs. Pain from hip OA is usually felt in the groin but can radiate to the anterior thigh or knee. Osteophytes from OA of the spine may cause radicular symptoms secondary to nerve root compression [6].

On physical examination, patients with OA often have bony enlargement and tenderness of the joint. Periarticular muscle spasm may be present. Range of motion (ROM) is sometimes limited. Locking of a joint during ROM can occur from loose bodies or fragments of cartilage in the joint space. Signs of mild inflammation, such as warmth or swelling, may be present around an affected joint. Evidence of severe inflammation is suspicious for other disorders, such as septic arthritis, gout, or pseudogout [6].

Crepitus is commonly felt on passive ROM of the knee. It is caused by the irregularity of the opposing cartilage surfaces. A varus deformity of the knee is often seen from medial compartment degeneration, but a valgus deformity is possible with lateral compartment involvement [6].

Bony enlargements called Heberden's nodes on the DIP joints and Bouchard's nodes on the PIP joints are frequently present in OA of the hand. These nodes may be painful, especially when they first develop, but are usually nontender after they are formed [6]. OA does not typically involve the metacarpophalangeal joints as rheumatoid arthritis does. Rheumatoid arthritis usually spares the DIP and first CMC joints commonly affected by OA.

OA is a clinical diagnosis. The majority of people with radiographic evidence of OA have no symptoms of OA [1]. Radiographs can help confirm OA when the diagnosis is uncertain from clinical examination. Osteophytes at the joint margin are a classic finding. Joint-space narrowing and subchondral bone sclerosis may be present in advanced disease. Erosions at the joint margins are not usually associated with OA; their presence suggests a more inflammatory type of arthritis [6].

Laboratory tests are not indicated except to evaluate for other diseases or to monitor potential adverse effects from pharmacotherapy. Healthy elderly patients may be positive for rheumatoid factor at low titers and often have modest elevations of erythrocyte sedimentation rate.

Therefore, these tests do not exclude OA and should be ordered only to confirm the presence of other disorders already suspected by history and physical examination [6].

TREATMENT

Nonpharmacologic Treatment

Numerous nonpharmacologic interventions have been proposed for the treatment of OA. The 2000 American College of Rheumatology (ACR) Subcommittee on Osteoarthritis Guidelines [7] describes nonpharmacologic modalities as the primary treatment of OA. These guidelines recommend that pharmacologic interventions be used only as adjuncts to nonpharmacologic measures. The evidence supporting nonpharmacologic therapies is sparse and is mainly limited to the treatment of knee OA.

Therapeutic Exercise (Grade of Recommendation: A for Knee Osteoarthritis; Level of Evidence: 1a)

A Cochrane review from 2001 [8] concluded that land-based therapeutic exercise seemed to reduce pain and improve function in symptomatic OA of the knee. Although the benefit was modest, it was comparable to the benefits reported with pharmacologic treatment. Group exercise classes and individual exercise programs had similar outcomes. There were insufficient data to make recommendations on the type of therapeutic exercise or on the frequency and duration of treatment. There were insufficient data on the effect of therapeutic exercise for symptomatic OA of the hip [8,9].

Weight Loss (Grade of Recommendation: B for Weight Loss Plus Exercise in Knee Osteoarthritis; Level of Evidence: 1b)

Observational studies have demonstrated an increased risk of knee OA in obese patients, particularly obese women, when compared with their non-obese counterparts [10,11]. There have been little data regarding the efficacy of weight loss for treatment of OA. In one observational study [12], women who had a decrease in body mass index of two units during a 10-year period demonstrated a 50% reduction in risk for developing new, symptomatic knee OA. A recent randomized control study (RCT) of older, overweight, and obese adults [13] evaluated the efficacy of exercise and dietary weight loss, separately and in combination, versus usual care for knee OA. Patients in the diet group and the diet-plus-exercise group lost an average of 5.7% and 4.9% of their body weight, respectively. Over 18 months, the diet-plus-exercise group showed statistically significant improvement in pain, self-reported physical function, stair-climb time, and 6-minute walk distance when compared with usual care. The exercise group had a statistically significant improvement in the 6-minute walk distance only. The diet-only group demonstrated no significant difference from usual care.

Ice Massage (Grade of Recommendation: D; Level of Evidence: 1a−)

A Cochrane review from 2003 [14] found that ice massage demonstrated a statistically significant benefit for ROM, function, and knee strength in patients with OA of the knee. The effectiveness for pain control was unclear. Ice therapy reduced swelling in patients with edema of the knee. However, due to the small number of RCTs and the heterogeneity of the studies, firm conclusions cannot be made.

Joint Bracing in Knee Osteoarthritis (Grade of Recommendation: A; Level of Evidence: 1b)

One RCT with 119 participants [9] found that valgus knee bracing was beneficial for disease-specific quality of life and function in OA of the knee. A smaller RCT of 14 participants [15] suggested that taping the patella medially reduced knee pain when the patellofemoral joint was involved.

Laterally Wedged Insoles (Grade of Recommendation: D; Level of Evidence 1b). Two RCTs and one nonrandomized controlled trial [16–18] evaluated laterally wedged insoles with subtalar strapping to correct varus deformities in patients with medial compartment knee OA. These studies demonstrated efficacy for the insoles, particularly in younger patients with a high lower-extremity lean body mass per body weight. Limitations of these trials are that they are from the same research group and included only Japanese women. Another RCT [19] evaluating laterally wedged insoles did not demonstrate a benefit for symptoms but showed a decrease in nonsteroidal anti-inflammatory drug (NSAID) consumption and better compliance in the treatment group. The patients in the treatment group had more severe OA, which restricts the interpretation of these findings. In summary, the limited evidence suggests a benefit of laterally wedged insoles in select patients with knee OA, but the data are insufficient to make a clear recommendation.

Acupuncture (Grade of Recommendation: D for Short-Term Pain Relief in Knee Ostearthritis; Level of Evidence: 1a−). A systematic review from 2001 [20] found good evidence from two high-quality RCTs that acupuncture improved pain in knee OA when compared with sham acupuncture. However, one high-quality RCT that used a different sham procedure did not demonstrate a significant difference. There was inconclusive evidence for improvement of function. The review found inconclusive evidence on the benefits of acupuncture when compared with physical therapy for pain or function. All of the studies included in the review used traditional Chinese medicine acupuncture without the supplemental herbs and individualized treatment that are usually part of this Chinese practice. Other acupuncture traditions have not been studied. It is difficult to determine if the limited benefits shown in these studies would be applicable to usual clinical practice.

Electrical Stimulation Therapy (Insufficient Evidence). Electrical stimulation to cartilage is thought to activate the production of proteoglycans, which are a major component of the cartilage matrix. This can be accomplished by direct placement of electrodes on the skin over the affected joint or by pulsed electromagnetic fields (PEMF). During PEMF therapy, the joint is inserted into a device that induces electrical current through magnetic impulses without direct contact to the skin. A Cochrane review from 2001 [21] found limited data suggesting statistically significant, but not clinically significant, benefits for electrical stimulation therapy. Further studies were recommended to clarify potential efficacy of this treatment modality.

Static magnets have been a popular complimentary therapy for the treatment of OA. The validity of studies has been limited by the ease of distinguishing a device containing true magnets from nonmagnetic placebos. A pilot study [22] using placebo-magnet sleeves designed to externally mimic the magnetic force of the therapeutic sleeve without producing a significant magnetic force in the knee joint suggested short-term efficacy of magnetic therapy for knee OA. A larger trial with longer follow-up may help to determine if static magnets are an effective therapy for OA.

Patient Education (Insufficient Evidence). A meta-analysis from 1996 [23] showed no statistically significant difference in pain or functional status between the patient education groups or control groups for patients with OA. A RCT in the United Kingdom [24] reported benefit with a self-management program for OA patients. However, a subsequent RCT [25], using the same program at primary care practices in the United States, did not demonstrate any benefit.

Pharmacologic Treatment

In many patients with OA, nonpharmacologic treatment is not adequate to control pain or improve functional status. Therefore, numerous pharmacologic therapies have been advocated for use in the management of OA. Table 1 provides a summary of the agents discussed in this section.

Acetaminophen (Grade of Recommendation: A for Short-Term Pain Relief; Level of Evidence: 1a)

A meta-analysis published in 2004 [26] confirmed the efficacy of acetaminophen in relieving pain due to OA. A Cochrane systematic review of 2002 [27] concluded that acetaminophen alleviated pain and improved patients' global assessment in the treatment of OA. Most of the studies used an acetaminophen dose of 4 g/d. In the RCTs reviewed, acetaminophen

TABLE 1.
Pharmacologic Treatments for Osteoarthritis

Pharmacologic Agent	Dosage	Grade of Recommendation[a]
Acetaminophen (Tylenol)	4000 mg/d	A
Oral NSAIDs	Various	A
Topical NSAIDs	Various	A
Topical capsaicin (Zostrix)	0.025% crm 4 times/d	A
Glucosamine sulfate	1500 mg/d	B
Chondroitin sulfate	1200 mg/d	B
S-adenosylmethionine	400–1200 mg/d	B
Avocado/soybean unsaponifiables	300 mg/d	B
Phytodolor	Various	Insufficient evidence
Opioids	Various	B
Intra-articular glucocorticoids for knee osteoarthritis	Various	A
Intra-articular hyaluronan (Hyalgan, Orthovisc, Synvisc)	Various	A

Abbreviation: NSAID, nonsteroidal anti-inflammatory drug.
[a] Recommendations are often limited to short-term treatment of pain. See text for details.

seemed to have an excellent safety profile; however, all of the studies were of relatively short duration.

There are observational data suggesting that therapeutic doses of acetaminophen can cause liver damage in persons with existing liver disease [9]. In addition, a case-control study [27] reported an increased risk of serious upper gastrointestinal (GI) events with higher doses (2–4 g/d) of acetaminophen. Acetaminophen seemed to potentiate the GI toxicity of NSAIDs. The relative risk of serious GI events was much higher in persons using 2 to 4 g/d of acetaminophen along with NSAIDs than reported with NSAID use alone. Although this adverse effect was rare and has not been observed in other studies, it raises a question about the long-term safety of high-dose acetaminophen use. Further studies are needed clarify this issue.

Acetaminophen Versus NSAIDs for First-Line Therapy. There has been ongoing debate about whether acetaminophen or NSAIDs should be first-line pharmacotherapy for OA. Previously, studies had not shown significant differences in pain relief between these two therapies [9]. Because acetaminophen had the advantages of low cost and minimal adverse effects, it was recommended as the first-line agent in the 1996 ACR guidelines. More recent evidence [27] suggests that NSAIDs are superior to acetaminophen for OA pain control, particularly in patients with more severe pain. Improvement in functional status seems to be similar with acetaminophen or NSAIDs. Consequently, the updated 2000 ACR guide-lines [7] state that NSAIDs could be considered as first-line pharmaco-therapy for OA instead of acetaminophen, especially in patients with moderate to severe pain.

A recent meta-analysis [28] comparing NSAIDs with acetaminophen reported that the difference in discontinuation due to adverse events between the two groups was not statistically significant. There was a trend for higher withdrawals in the NSAID groups. This was especially evident with the high-dose NSAID groups. Because the overall number of dropouts was small and because the studies provided limited data about reasons for withdrawal, it is difficult to draw conclusions from these results.

Oral NSAIDs (Grade of Recommendation: A for Short-Term Pain Relief; Level of Evidence: 1a)

Systematic reviews of RCTs [9,29,30] found evidence that NSAIDs reduce OA pain when compared with placebo in short-term studies. These reviews found no significant difference in efficacy between different NSAIDs. The differences reported in some studies were not clinically significant because nonequivalent doses were used. COX-2 inhibitors seem to have similar efficacy as nonselective NSAIDs. Therefore, the choice of NSAID should be based on other factors, such as safety and cost [31,32].

Nonselective NSAIDs have shown the potential for serious GI, renal, and cardiovascular toxicity. Risk factors for NSAID-induced GI toxicity include age ≥65, history of peptic ulcer disease or upper GI bleeding, use of glucocorticoids or anticoagulants, and presence of comorbid conditions. Risk factors for NSAID-induced renal failure in patients with renal disease include age ≥65, hypertension, congestive heart failure, and use of diuretics or ACE inhibitors. Studies have shown that GI adverse events occur more commonly with nonselective NSAIDs than with acetaminophen. When all NSAIDs (nonselective and COX-2 inhibitors) were compared with acetaminophen, the difference in GI adverse effects was not statistically significant [27]. This finding suggests that COX-2 inhibitors may have an incidence of GI toxicity comparable to acetaminophen.

Two meta-analyses [33,34] have ranked the risk of GI toxicity with various nonselective NSAIDs. The rankings for these NSAIDs are summarized in Table 2. NSAIDs that are not available in the United States have been excluded. The first meta-analysis [33] pooled data from epidemiologic studies, whereas the second meta-analysis [34] combined data from RCTs and controlled-cohort studies. Most of the studies included in these analyses used low doses of ibuprofen. The earlier meta-analysis [33] included studies with low doses of diclofenac. If the full anti-inflammatory doses of ibuprofen and diclofenac were used, their GI risk might have been higher. The reason for the significant difference in risk with piroxicam is unclear.

Although COX-2 inhibitors seem to have a lower risk of GI toxicity, rofecoxib has been found to be associated with an increased risk of

TABLE 2.
Ranking of Selected Nonsteroidal Anti-inflammatory Drugs According to Reported Gastrointestinal Toxicity[a]

	Henry et al [33]	Richy et al [34]
Ibuprofen (Advil, Motrin)	1/8	1/6
Meloxicam (Mobic)	—	2/6
Aspirin	2/8	—
Diclofenac (Voltaren, Cataflam)	3/8	4/6
Sulindac (Clinoril)	4/8	—
Naproxen (Naprosyn, Naprelan)	5/8	5/6
Indomethacin (Indocin)	6/8	6/6
Piroxicam (Feldene)	7/8	3/6
Ketoprofen (Orudis, Oruvail)	8/8	—

[a] Least toxic = 1.

cardiovascular events [35,36], resulting in its withdrawal from the market on September 30, 2004. It is not clear whether this is a class effect for all COX-2 inhibitors. Concomitant use of aspirin may reduce the risk of cardiovascular events but may eliminate or decrease the GI advantage of COX-2 inhibitors.

Prevention of NSAID-Induced Gastrointestinal Toxicity. Several strategies have been studied for the prevention of NSAID-induced GI toxicity. Table 3 summarizes these strategies. A Cochrane review from 2002 [37] concluded that misoprostol, proton pump inhibitors (PPIs), and double-dose H2 receptor antagonists (H2RAs) were effective at preventing NSAID-induced gastric and duodenal ulcers detected by endoscope. Standard-dose H2RAs were effective at preventing duodenal ulcers only. Misoprostol 800 mg/d was the only agent shown to reduce the risk of serious complications such as perforation, hemorrhage, or obstruction.

Endoscopic ulcers can be detected in up to 40% of chronic NSAID users, but as many as 85% of these never become clinically apparent. Therefore, the clinical significance of endoscopic ulcers is questionable. A systematic review from 2004 [38] used symptomatic ulcers or serious GI complications (upper GI bleed, hemorrhagic erosion, perforation, or pyloric obstruction) as primary outcomes in assessing strategies for the prevention of NSAID-induced GI toxicity. It included COX-2 inhibitors as a strategy for reducing GI complications. This review found that using misoprostol in combination with nonselective NSAIDs and possibly using COX-2 inhibitors alone reduced the risk of serious GI complications. Misoprostol, COX-2 inhibitors, and possibly PPIs reduced the risk of symptomatic ulcers. There were insufficient data to draw conclusions about H2RAs for any of the primary outcomes. All of the strategies, including H2RAs, reduced the incidence of endoscopic ulcers.

In summary, misoprostol 800 mg/d is the only agent shown to be effective in preventing symptomatic ulcers and serious GI complications.

TABLE 3.
Strategies for Prevention of NSAID induced GI toxicity (LOE 1a)

Agents Used with Nonselective NSAIDs	Dosage	Reduces Symptomatic Ulcers?	Reduces Serious GI Complications?[a]	Reduces Endoscopic Gastric and Duodenal Ulcers?	Reduces Endoscopic Duodenal Ulcers Only?
Misoprostol	800 mg/d	Yes	Yes	Yes	—
H2RAs	Standard dose	Insufficient data	Insufficient data	No	Yes
H2RAs	Double dose	Insufficient data	Insufficient data	Yes	—
PPIs	Various	Yes?[b]	Insufficient data	Yes	—
COX-2 inhibitors alone	Various	Yes	Yes?[b]	Yes	—

Abbreviations: GI, gastrointestinal; H2RA, H2 receptor antagonist; LOE, level of evidence; NSAID, nonsteroidal anti-inflammatory drug; PPI, proton pump inhibitor.

[a] Serious GI complications include upper GI bleed, hemorrhagic erosion, perforation, pyloric obstruction.

[b] ? Denotes that apparent reduction of events was lost on sensitivity analysis.

Data from Rostrum A, Dube C, Wells G, et al. Prevention of NSAID-induced gastroduodenal ulcers. In: The Cochrane Library, issue 3. Chichester, UK: John Wiley & Sons; 2004; and Hooper L, Brown TJ, Elliott R, et al. The effectiveness of five strategies for the prevention of gastrointestinal toxicity induced by non-steroidal anti-inflammatory drugs: systematic review. BMJ 2004;329:948.

However, its frequent side effects, such as diarrhea and abdominal pain, limit its use. Lower doses have fewer side effects but have demonstrated decreased efficacy in the prevention of endoscopic ulcers. The effectiveness of lower doses for preventing serious GI complications is unknown but is assumed to be significantly decreased [37]. There are much less data on the other strategies. COX-2 inhibitors seemed to reduce the risk of symptomatic ulcers and possibly serious GI complications, but concerns about the cardiovascular risk of these agents may limit their use. Further studies are needed to clarify the effectiveness of PPIs and H2RAs in the prevention of the more clinically significant NSAID-induced adverse effects, such as symptomatic ulcers and other serious GI complications.

Topical NSAIDs (Grade of Recommendation: A for Short-Term Pain Relief; Level of Evidence: 1a)

A systematic review and subsequent RCTs [31] have found that topical NSAIDs reduce chronic musculoskeletal pain when compared with placebo in short-term studies. There was insufficient evidence to compare typical versus oral preparations of the same NSAID. There was also insufficient evidence to compare typical NSAIDs with other therapies, such as acetaminophen or other local treatments.

Topical Capsaicin (Grade of Recommendation: A for Short-Term Pain Relief; Level of Evidence: 1b)

A meta-analysis of three RCTs [39] and a subsequent RCT [9] found capsaicin cream to be effective for reducing OA pain when compared with placebo. Repeated application of capsaicin is thought to cause desensitization of pain fibers after an initial period of increased sensitivity. Local skin irritation is a common side effect resulting from this initial sensitivity. There are insufficient data to compare capsaicin with any other treatment.

Glucosamine (Grade of Recommendation: B; Level of Evidence: 1a−)

Glucosamine is a natural substance derived from animal products. In vitro studies have concluded that glucosamine stimulates proteoglycan synthesis in articular cartilage, theoretically rebuilding damaged cartilage. This hypothesis might explain why glucosamine seems to take several weeks to demonstrate any therapeutic effect. Animal models have shown a mild anti-inflammatory effect. There is no conclusive evidence of any of these findings in humans [40].

Two systematic reviews [40,41] concluded that glucosamine was safe and effective for treating symptoms of OA in short-term trials. Glucosamine sulfate 1500 mg/d was the most common preparation used. The Cochrane review [40] included trials comparing glucosamine with

NSAIDs and with placebo. In the NSAID trials, glucosamine was found to be equivalent or superior to each NSAID studied. The authors of the second review [41] noted that trial quality and publication bias may have contributed to the moderate to large effect reported for glucosamine. However, even a small benefit may be significant due to the safety of glucosamine. The Cochrane review noted that most of the studies used a preparation of glucosamine sulfate from the same manufacturer. It is unclear whether preparations from other manufacturers would have the same benefit. The only RCT in the Cochrane review that did not demonstrate superior efficacy for glucosamine when compared with placebo was the only study that used glucosamine hydrochloride rather than glucosamine sulfate. The review found insufficient evidence to comment on the long-term effectiveness and safety of glucosamine. Subsequent RCTs have had less consistent results [9]. There is one RCT [42] in which glucosamine significantly reduced mean joint space narrowing (by radiographic measurements) over 3 years compared with placebo. This is the first preliminary evidence that glucosamine may be a disease-modifying agent in the treatment of OA, as hypothesized from in vitro and animal studies.

Chondroitin Sulfate (Grade of Recommendation: B; Level of Evidence: 1a−)

Chondroitin sulfate is a natural substance derived from animal products. Like glucosamine, it is thought to stimulate proteoglycan synthesis in articular cartilage. There is no evidence from human studies to support this theoretical role in cartilage repair. The most common dosage is 1200 mg/d, although doses have varied in trials.

A systematic review [41] evaluated the effectiveness of chondroitin sulfate in the treatment of OA. It reported moderate to large beneficial effects. This review cautioned that, as with glucosamine, the effect was likely exaggerated by trial quality and publication bias. Another meta-analysis of RCTs [43] concluded that chondroitin sulfate may be beneficial in the treatment of OA. The authors stated that further studies of longer duration and with larger numbers of patients were needed to confirm chondroitin's effectiveness. Subsequent RCTs have had mixed results [9]. One RCT comparing chondroitin with a NSAID found that the NSAID was more effective at 30 days, but at 60 days chondroitin was more effective. If this finding is confirmed, it would be consistent with the hypothesis that agents such as chondroitin and glucosamine help to rebuild articular cartilage. This mechanism of action could explain why these agents seem to possess a slower onset of action but better long-term efficacy.

There are insufficient data to compare the effectiveness of the combination of glucosamine and chondroitin sulfate with either agent alone [9]. The Glucosamine/Chondroitin Arthritis Intervention Trial is a placebo-controlled RCT designed to compare glucosamine alone, chondroitin alone, the combination of glucosamine and chondroitin, and celecoxib in the treatment of OA of the knee. Changes in joint space width are one of the outcomes measured. Scheduled completion of this trial is November 2005. The results of this trial may help to clarify the efficacy and mechanism of action of glucosamine and chondroitin sulfate.

S-adenosylmethionine (Grade of Recommendation: B; Level of Evidence: 1a−)

S-adenosylmethionine (SAMe) is a naturally occurring compound found throughout the body. In vitro studies of SAMe have demonstrated an increase of proteoglycan synthesis in articular cartilage, suggesting an ability to repair damaged cartilage. Other mechanisms of action, such as decreasing inflammation and providing analgesia, have been proposed. SAMe seems to possess serotonergic activity and has been shown to decrease depression [44,45].

A meta-analysis of RCTs from 2002 [44] concluded that SAMe seemed to be as effective as NSAIDs in reducing pain and improving function in patients with OA. Oral doses from 400 to 1200 mg/d were used. Most of the trials were only 1 month in duration. Besides the absence of long-term data, the authors noted that they could not exclude SAMe's antidepressant qualities as a factor contributing to its apparent efficacy. A subsequent RCT [45] compared 1200 mg/d SAMe with celecoxib 200 mg/d for treatment of knee OA. It was a double-blind, cross-over study with each phase lasting 8 weeks and a 1-week washout period between phases. In this study, SAMe demonstrated similar efficacy as celecoxib; however, SAMe had a slower onset of action, requiring nearly 1 month to achieve the same benefit as celecoxib. This trial evaluated the possibility that antidepressant activity might affect the results. The authors concluded that the benefits for pain and function were independent of any antidepressant effect. Consistent with previous trials, side-effects of SAMe were mild and significantly less than those of NSAIDs. A problem in this study was that the SAMe preparation had lost 50% of its potency at one point in the trial. A new batch of SAMe was substituted, allowing the trial to continue. Nonetheless, this occurrence highlights the concern about the stability of SAMe preparations. As with other dietary supplements, the precise amount of active ingredient contained in commercial preparations can vary.

Although the data suggest that SAMe is an effective therapy for OA, further studies are needed to verify this finding in larger trials of longer duration. Clarification of the optimal dose is necessary.

Avocado/Soybean Unsaponifiables (Grade of Recommendation: B; Level of Evidence: 1a)

A Cochrane review from 2001 [46] investigated data on various herbal therapies used to treat OA. The authors concluded that there was convincing evidence for the use of avocado/soybean unsaponifiables (ASUs). Two RCTs using a mixture of one third avocado and two thirds soybean unsaponifiables were evaluated. The outcomes were improvement of pain and function, decrease of NSAID use, and continued benefit after discontinuation of ASUs. The active ingredients of this compound have not been identified. In vitro studies have suggested that ASUs may assist in the repair of damaged articular cartilage. This may explain the delayed onset of action (up to 2 months) of ASUs [46,47].

A second systematic review from 2001 [47] concluded that data from the ASU studies was promising. However, the authors point out that both RCTs originated from the same research group. Therefore, further studies by other groups are required to confirm these findings.

Phytodolor (Insufficient Evidence)

Phytodolor is an herbal mixture proposed to have anti-inflammatory properties. It was evaluated as a treatment for musculoskeletal pain in a systematic review from 2000 [48]. Inflammatory and noninflammatory conditions were included in this review. The author concluded that phytodolor was a safe and effective treatment. Heterogeneity between the trials makes the results difficult to interpret. A systematic review from 2001 [47] evaluated phytodolor as a treatment specifically for OA. These authors also concluded that phytodolor demonstrated effectiveness for pain and function. Problems with the validity assessments and potential publication bias bring these conclusions into question.

Opioids (Grade of Recommendation: B; Level of Evidence: 1b)

When OA pain is not controlled with other strategies or when patients cannot tolerate other pharmacologic therapies, opioids may be considered for the treatment of OA. The significant adverse effects (particularly in elderly patients), the development of tolerance, the risk of dependence, and the strict regulation of these controlled substances contribute to the reluctance of providers to use opioids in the treatment of chronic pain. Few RCTs have evaluated opioids specifically for the treatment of OA. Two RCTs [49,50] evaluating codeine in combination with acetaminophen or ibuprofen found that the codeine combinations were more effective for treatment of OA pain than acetaminophen or ibuprofen alone. However, there was a high incidence of adverse effects with subsequent withdrawal from the study in the codeine groups. Oxycodone has demonstrated efficacy for OA pain in RCTs [51,52]. Other opioids, such as hydrocodone, morphine, and hydromorphone, have not been adequately studied in OA. Their presumed benefit is based on extrapolations from chronic pain trials. Generally, the controlled release preparations of opioids are associated with fewer side effects.

Tramadol is a centrally acting analgesic with opioid and non-opioid activity. It is not a controlled substance and does not seem to cause tolerance or dependence. GI and other central nervous system side effects are similar to those of opioids, except that tramadol does not seem to cause respiratory depression [53]. This improved side-effect profile, when compared with opioids, has made tramadol an attractive alternative in the treatment of pain. Three recent RCTs have evaluated tramadol for the treatment of OA. The first study [54] evaluated tramadol versus placebo for breakthrough pain in patients with OA who were on stable NSAID therapy. Tramadol demonstrated a statistically significant benefit for pain at rest and for patients' overall assessment of therapy. The second study [55] assessed whether tramadol 200 mg/d could allow patients to lower their dose of naproxen without compromising pain relief. Results showed that, in patients who had pain relief with 1000 mg/d of naproxen, adding tramadol 200 mg/d permitted significant decreases in the naproxen dosage without affecting pain control. The third study [56] compared extended-release tramadol with placebo in patients with moderate to severe chronic OA pain. Tramadol extended-release (ER) demonstrated statistically significant benefits for all of the outcomes, including pain and function.

Intra-articular Glucocorticoid Injection of the Knee (Grade of Recommendation: A for Short-Term Pain Relief; Level of Evidence: 1a)

One systematic review and one subsequent RCT [9] demonstrated pain relief, lasting 1 to 4 weeks, after glucocorticoid injection of the knee when compared with placebo. Concerns about the possible risk of articular cartilage damage with repeated glucocorticoid injections usually limit the use of this therapy to every 3 or 4 months for any given joint.

Intra-articular Hyaluronic Acid Injection of the Knee (Grade of Recommendation: A for Short-Term Treatment; Level of Evidence: 1a)

Hyaluronic acid (HA) is a component of human synovial fluid that increases its viscosity. OA is associated with a decrease of HA content in the synovial fluid [4]. It has been theorized that intra-articular viscosupplementation with HA can modify disease progression in knee OA. There is insufficient evidence to support this theory [57]. Two systematic reviews [9,58] have evaluated the efficacy of intra-articular HA in the treatment of knee OA. Both reviews concluded that intra-articular HA has a greater effect on pain and function in the short term than placebo. A series of HA injections were usually performed over several weeks. Generally, it took more than 1 month to demonstrate benefit with HA, but the effects lasted 3 to 6 months. Adverse effects were rare. Higher-molecular-weight preparations, such as Hylan G-F 20 (Synvisc), seem to be more effective than lower-molecular-weight preparations [57,58]. The benefit from the placebo saline injections was high in some of the studies. In addition, there is insufficient evidence to determine whether simple aspiration of the knee might be as effective as injection [9].

Surgical Treatment

There are no evidence-based criteria regarding indications for the referral of a patient with OA for surgical treatment. Most consensus statements recommend that patients who continue to have severe pain and functional limitation from OA of the knee or hip, despite maximal conservative therapy, should be referred to an orthopedic surgeon for consideration of surgical treatment [7,57,59,60]. Several of the surgical options for OA treatment are discussed below.

Arthroscopic Debridement (Not Recommended; Level of Evidence: 1b)

In one RCT [61], there was no benefit from arthroscopic debridement or lavage versus a placebo procedure in patients with knee OA. This suggests that the subjective pain relief reported from arthroscopic debridement is due to a placebo effect. It is unclear whether arthroscopic debridement would be more efficacious if performed in select patients, such as younger patients with chondral or meniscal lesions amenable to debridement.

Osteotomy (Grade of Recommendation: B for Medial Unicompartmental Knee Osteoarthritis; Level of Evidence: 1b)

The degenerative changes of knee OA can alter joint mechanics. Medial compartment degeneration causes a varus deformity, and lateral compartment degeneration causes a valgus deformity. These deformities shift the weight-bearing stress toward the affected compartment of the knee. When knee OA is limited to the medial compartment, high tibial osteotomies are sometimes performed. The rationale for this procedure is to correct the varus deformity and redistribute the weight-bearing stress of the joint [62]. Two RCTs comparing osteotomy with unicompartmental knee replacement found similar functional outcomes in the two groups [9]. No RCTs were found comparing high tibial osteotomies with conservative therapy for knee OA. Osteotomies can be performed for lateral unicompartmental knee OA and for hip OA, but there is insufficient evidence regarding these procedures.

Total Hip Replacement/Arthroplasty (Grade of Recommendation: A; Level of Evidence: 1a–)

A systematic review of RCTs and observational studies concluded that hip replacement is effective for at least 10 years [9]. A recent systematic review of cohort studies [63] evaluated the health-related quality of life after total hip and total knee arthroplasty. Both procedures resulted in substantial improvements in physical health, including pain and function. Improvements in mental and social health were more modest. Total hip replacement improved function to a greater extent than did total knee replacement. Primary surgery had better outcomes than revision. Age did not seem to be a significant factor.

Knee Replacement/Arthroplasty (Grade of Recommendation: B; Level of Evidence: 2a)

Systematic reviews of primarily cohort studies have concluded that knee replacement improves pain and function in patients with knee OA [9]. If more than one compartment is involved, total knee replacement is generally recommended. In patients with OA of only the medial knee compartment, several options exist including osteotomy and unicompartmental knee replacement. One RCT found that unicompartmental knee replacement was more effective than total knee replacement in patients with OA of the medial knee compartment [9].

A systematic review of cohort trials [63] determined that total knee replacement resulted in significant improvements in health-related quality of life. However, the benefits were less pronounced than those resulting from hip replacement.

Key Points

- OA is the most common form of arthritis, causing significant pain, functional impairment, and disability.
- Risk factors for OA include advanced age, female gender, genetic predisposition, joint injury, and obesity.
- OA is characterized by the progressive breakdown of articular cartilage, associated with inflammation, osteophyte formation, and joint deformity.
- Nonpharmacologic interventions, such as therapeutic exercise alone (grade of recommendation A), joint bracing (grade of recommendation A), and exercise plus dietary weight loss (grade of recommendation B), should be considered in patients with knee osteoarthritis.
- Pharmacologic therapies with a grade of recommendation A for short-term treatment of OA include acetaminophen, oral and topical NSAIDs, topical capsaicin, and intra-articular glucocorticoid (A) or hyaluronic acid (A) injections of the knee.
- Pharmacologic therapies with a grade of recommendation B for short-term treatment of OA include glucosamine sulfate, chondroitin sulfate, SAMe, ASUs, and opioids.
- Animal and in vitro studies suggest that glucosamine, chondroitin sulfate, SAMe, ASU, and intra-articular hyaluronic acid act as disease-modifying agents rather than analgesics. Further human studies are needed to confirm this hypothesis.
- There are primarily observational data supporting the use of hip and knee replacement for the treatment of osteoarthritis. Evidence regarding the timing of surgery and selection of patients is lacking.

ACKNOWLEDGMENTS

I would like to thank Dr. James Glass for his assistance in obtaining reference articles used for this publication.

References

[1] Lawrence RC, Helmick CG, Arnett FC, et al. Estimates of the prevalence of arthritis and selected musculoskeletal disorders in the United States. Arthritis Rheum 1998;41: 778–99.

[2] CDC. Prevalence of disabilities and associated health conditions among adults: United States, 1999. MMWR 2001;50:120–5.

[3] Sinkov V, Cymet T. Osteoarthritis: understanding the pathophysiology, genetics, and treatments. J Natl Med Assoc 2003;95:475–82.

[4] Fife R. Osteoarthritis: A. Epidemiology, pathology and pathogenesis. In: Klippel JH, editor. Primer on the rheumatic diseases. 11th edition. Atlanta: The Arthritis Foundation; 1997. p. 216–7.

[5] Martel-Pelletier J. Pathophysiology of osteoarthritis. Osteoarthritis Cartilage 2004;12(Suppl A):S31–3.

[6] Hochberg M. Osteoarthritis: B. Clinical features and treatment. In: Klippel JH, editor. Primer on the rheumatic diseases. 11th edition. Atlanta: The Arthritis Foundation; 1997. p. 218–21.

[7] Recommendations for the medical management of osteoarthritis of the hip and knee: 2000 update. American College of Rheumatology Subcommittee on Osteoarthritis Guidelines. Arthritis Rheum 2000;43:1905–15.

[8] Fransen M, McConnell S, Bell M. Exercise for osteoarthritis of the hip or knee. In: The Cochrane Library, Issue 3. Chichester, UK: John Wiley and Sons; 2004.

[9] Scott D, Smith C, Lohmander S, et al. Osteoarthritis. Clin Evid 2004;11:1560–88.

[10] Felson DT. Does excess weight cause osteoarthritis and, if so, why? Ann Rheum Dis 1996;55:668–70.

[11] Nevitt MC. Obesity outcomes in disease management: clinical outcomes for osteoarthritis. Obes Res 2002;10(Suppl 1):33S–7S.

[12] Felson DT, Zhang Y, Anthony JM, et al. Weight loss reduces the risk for symptomatic knee osteoarthritis in women. The Framingham Study. Ann Intern Med 1992;116:535–9.

[13] Messier SP, Loeser RF, Miller GD, et al. Exercise and dietary weight loss in overweight and obese older adults with knee osteoarthritis: the Arthritis, Diet, and Activity Promotion Trial. Arthritis Rheum 2004;50:1501–10.

[14] Brosseau L, Yonge KA, Robinson V, et al. Thermotherapy for treatment of osteoarthritis. In: The Cochrane Library, issue 3. Chichester, UK: John Wiley and Sons; 2004.

[15] Cushnaghan J, McCarthy C, Dieppe P. Taping the patella medially: a new treatment for osteoarthritis of the knee joint? BMJ 1994;308:753–5.

[16] Toda Y, Segal N. Usefulness of an insole with subtalar strapping for analgesia in patients with medial compartment osteoarthritis of the knee. Arthritis Rheum 2002;47:468–73.

[17] Toda Y, Segal N, Kato A, et al. Correlation between body composition and efficacy of lateral wedged insoles for medial compartment osteoarthritis of the knee. J Rheumatol 2002;29:541–5.

[18] Toda Y, Segal N, Kato A, et al. Effect of a novel insole on the subtalar joint of patients with medial compartment osteoarthritis of the knee. J Rheumatol 2001;28:2705–10.

[19] Maillefert JF, Hudry C, Baron G, et al. Laterally elevated wedged insoles in the treatment of medial knee osteoarthritis: a prospective randomized controlled study. Osteoarthritis Cartilage 2001;9:738–45.

[20] Ezzo J, Hadhazy V, Birch S, et al. Acupuncture for osteoarthritis of the knee: a systematic review. Arthritis Rheum 2001;44:819–25.

[21] Hulme J, Robinson V, DeBie R, et al. Electromagnetic fields for the treatment of osteoarthritis. In: The Cochrane Library, issue 3. Chichester, UK: John Wiley and Sons; 2004.

[22] Wolsko PM, Eisenberg DM, Simon LS, et al. Double-blind placebo-controlled trial of static magnets for the treatment of osteoarthritis of the knee: results of a pilot study. Altern Ther Health Med 2004;10:36–43.

[23] Superio-Cabuslay E, Ward MM, Lorig KR. Patient education interventions in osteoarthritis and rheumatoid arthritis: a meta-analytic comparison with nonsteroidal antiinflammatory drug treatment. Arthritis Care Res 1996;9:292–301.

[24] Barlow JH, Turner AP, Wright CC. A randomized controlled study of the Arthritis Self-Management Programme in the UK. Health Educ Res 2000;15:665–80.

[25] Solomon DH, Warsi A, Brown-Stevenson T, et al. Does self-management education benefit all populations with arthritis? A randomized controlled trial in a primary care physician network. J Rheumatol 2002;29:362–8.

[26] Zhang W, Jones A, Doherty M. Does paracetamol (acetaminophen) reduce the pain of osteoarthritis? A meta-analysis of randomised controlled trials. Ann Rheum Dis 2004;63: 901–7.

[27] Towheed TE, Judd MJ, Hochberg MC, et al. Acetaminophen for osteoarthritis. In: The Cochrane Library, issue 3. Chichester, UK: John Wiley and Sons; 2004.

[28] Lee C, Straus WL, Balshaw R, et al. A comparison of the efficacy and safety of nonsteroidal antiinflammatory agents versus acetaminophen in the treatment of osteoarthritis: a meta-analysis. Arthritis Rheum 2004;51:746–54.

[29] Towheed T, Shea B, Wells G, et al. Analgesia and non-aspirin, non-steroidal anti-inflammatory drugs for osteoarthritis of the hip. Cochrane Database Syst Rev 1997;4: CD000517.

[30] Watson MC, Brookes ST, Kirwan JR, et al. Non-aspirin, non-steroidal anti-inflammatory drugs for osteoarthritis of the knee. Cochrane Database Syst Rev 1997;1:CD000142.

[31] Gotzche P. Non-steroidal anti-inflammatory drugs. Clin Evid 2004;11:1551–9.

[32] Deeks JJ, Smith LA, Bradley MD. Efficacy, tolerability, and upper gastrointestinal safety of celecoxib for treatment of osteoarthritis and rheumatoid arthritis: systematic review of randomised controlled trials. BMJ 2002;325:619–23.

[33] Henry D, Lim LL, Garcia Rodriguez LA, et al. Variability in risk of gastrointestinal complications with individual non-steroidal anti-inflammatory drugs: results of a collaborative meta-analysis. BMJ 1996;312:1563–6.

[34] Richy F, Bruyere O, Ethgan O, et al. Time dependent risk of gastrointestinal complications induced by non-steroidal anti-inflammatory drug use: a consensus statement using a meta-analytic approach. Ann Rheum Dis 2004;63:759–66.

[35] Mukherjee D, Nissen SE, Topol EJ. Risk of cardiovascular events associated with selective COX-2 inhibitors. JAMA 2001;286:954–9.

[36] Merck announces voluntary worldwide withdrawal of Vioxx. Available at: www.merck.com/newsroompress_releases/product/200_0930.html. Accessed November 6, 2004.

[37] Rostrum A, Dube C, Wells G, et al. Prevention of NSAID-induced gastroduodenal ulcers. In: The Cochrane Library, issue 3. Chichester, UK: John Wiley & Sons; 2004.

[38] Hooper L, Brown TJ, Elliott RA, et al. The effectiveness of five strategies for the prevention of gastrointestinal toxicity induced by non-steroidal anti-inflammatory drugs: systematic review. BMJ 2004;329:948.

[39] Zhang WY, Li Wan Po A. The effectiveness of topically applied capsaicin: a meta-analysis. Eur J Clin Pharmacol 1994;46:517–22.

[40] Towheed TE, Anastassiades TP, Shea B, et al. Glucosamine therapy for treating osteoarthritis. In: The Cochrane Library, issue 3. Chichester, UK: John Wiley and Sons; 2004.

[41] McAlindon TE, LaValley MP, Gulin JP, et al. Glucosamine and chondroitin for treatment of osteoarthritis: a systematic quality assessment and meta-analysis. JAMA 2000;283: 1469–75.

[42] Pavelka K, Gatterova J, Olejarova M, et al. Glucosamine sulfate use and delay of progression of knee osteoarthritis: a 3-year, randomized, placebo-controlled, double-blind study. Arch Intern Med 2002;162:2113–23.

[43] Leeb BF, Schweitzer H, Montag K, et al. A metaanalysis of chondroitin sulfate in the treatment of osteoarthritis. J Rheumatol 2000;27:205–11.

[44] Soeken KL, Lee WL, Bausell RB, et al. Safety and efficacy of S-adenosylmethionine (SAMe) for osteoarthritis. J Fam Pract 2002;51:425–30.

[45] Najm WI, Reinsch S, Hoehler F, et al. S-adenosyl methionine (SAMe) versus celecoxib for the treatment of osteoarthritis symptoms: a double-blind cross-over trial. BMC Musculoskelet Disord 2004;5:6.

[46] Little CV, Parsons T. Herbal therapy for treating osteoarthritis. In: The Cochrane Library, issue 3. Chichester, UK: John Wiley and Sons; 2004.

[47] Long L, Soeken K, Ernst E. Herbal medicines for the treatment of osteoarthritis: a systematic review. Rheumatology (Oxford) 2001;40:779–93.

[48] Ernst E. The efficacy of Phytodolor for the treatment of musculoskeletal pain: a systematic review of randomized clinical trials. Natur Med Online 2000;3.

[49] Kjaersgaard-Andersen P, Nafei A, Skov O, et al. Codeine plus paracetamol versus paracetamol in longer-term treatment of chronic pain due to osteoarthritis of the hip: a randomized, double-blind, multi-centre study. Pain 1990;43:309–18.

[50] Quiding H, Grimstad J, Rusten K, et al. Ibuprofen plus codeine, ibuprofen, and placebo in a single- and multidose cross-over comparison for coxarthrosis pain. Pain 1992;50:303–7.

[51] Roth SH, Fleischmann RM, Burch FX, et al. Around-the-clock, controlled-release oxycodone therapy for osteoarthritis-related pain: placebo-controlled trial and long-term evaluation. Arch Intern Med 2000;160:853–60.

[52] Lipman AG. Treatment of chronic pain in osteoarthritis: do opioids have a clinical role? Curr Rheumatol Rep 2001;3:513–9.

[53] Katz WA. Pharmacology and clinical experience with tramadol in osteoarthritis. Drugs 1996;52(Suppl 3):39–47.

[54] Roth SH. Efficacy and safety of tramadol HCl in breakthrough musculoskeletal pain attributed to osteoarthritis. J Rheumatol 1998;25:1358–63.

[55] Schnitzer TJ, Kamin M, Olson WH. Tramadol allows reduction of naproxen dose among patients with naproxen-responsive osteoarthritis pain: a randomized, double-blind, placebo-controlled study. Arthritis Rheum 1999;42:1370–7.

[56] Babul N, Noveck R, Chipman H, et al. Efficacy and safety of extended-release, once-daily tramadol in chronic pain: a randomized 12-week clinical trial in osteoarthritis of the knee. J Pain Symptom Manage 2004;28:59–71.

[57] Jordan KM, Arden NK, Doherty M, et al. Standing Committee for International Clinical Studies Including Therapeutic Trials ESCISIT. EULAR Recommendations 2003: an evidence based approach to the management of knee osteoarthritis: report of a Task Force of the Standing Committee for International Clinical Studies Including Therapeutic Trials (ESCISIT). Ann Rheum Dis 2003;62:1145–55.

[58] Espallargues M, Pons JM. Efficacy and safety of viscosupplementation with Hylan G-F 20 for the treatment of knee osteoarthritis: a systematic review. Int J Technol Assess Health Care 2003;19:41–56.

[59] American Academy of Orthopaedic Surgeons. AAOS clinical guideline on osteoarthritis of the knee (phase II). Rosemont (IL): American Academy of Orthopaedic Surgeons; 2003, p. 15.

[60] Zhang W, Doherty M, Arden N, et al. EULAR evidence based recommendations for the management of hip osteoarthritis: report of a task force of the EULAR Standing Committee for International Clinical Studies Including Therapeutics (ESCISIT). Ann Rheum Dis 2004 [epub ahead of print].

[61] Moseley JB, O'Malley K, Petersen NJ, et al. A controlled trial of arthroscopic surgery for osteoarthritis of the knee. N Engl J Med 2002;347:81–8.

[62] Gidwani S, Fairbank A. The orthopaedic approach to managing osteoarthritis of the knee. BMJ 2004;329:1220–4.

[63] Ethgen O, Bruyere O, Richy F, et al. Health-related quality of life in total hip and total knee arthroplasty: a qualitative and systematic review of the literature. J Bone Joint Surg Am 2004;86-A:963–74.

Address reprint requests to

Gina Gill Glass, MD
216 Sherbrooke Dr.
Newport News, VA 23602

e-mail: gmgill@pol.net

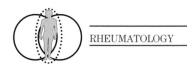
FIBROMYALGIA AND DIFFUSE MYALGIA

James M. Gill, MD, MPH, and Anna Quisel, MD

PREVALENCE, PRESENTATION, AND PROGRESSION OF THE PATIENT WITH FIBROMYALGIA

Chronic pain is one of the most common complaints encountered by primary care clinicians. Often, patients present not with well localized pain but with diffuse and nonspecific myalgias. Fibromyalgia is the most common etiology for this type of pain. In community-based studies, 2% [1] and 1.2% to 6.2% of school-age children screened positive for fibromyalgia [2–4]. Women and girls are at higher risk than males, and risk increases with age, peaking between 55 and 79 years [1,5].

Persons suffering from fibromyalgia most commonly complain of widespread pain. The pain is usually bilateral and is usually worse in the neck and trunk [6]. Additional symptoms include fatigue, waking unrefreshed, morning stiffness, paresthesias, and headaches [6–12]. Compared with patients with other rheumatologic conditions, persons with fibromyalgia more often suffer from comorbid conditions [13], including chronic fatigue syndrome, migraine headaches, irritable bowel syndrome, irritable bladder symptoms, temporomandibular joint syndrome, myofascial pain syndrome, restless leg syndrome, and affective disorders [13–15].

Fibromyalgia can cause significant morbidity [1,16,17]. Patients with fibromyalgia require an average of 2.7 drugs at any time for fibromyalgia-related symptoms and have an average of 10 outpatient visits per year, with one hospitalization every 3 years [13]. Fibromyalgia has been associated with higher rates of osteoporosis [18]. Patients with fibromyalgia have higher rates of surgery, including hysterectomies, appendectomies, back/neck surgery, and carpal tunnel surgery, compared with patients with other

From the Department of Family and Community Medicine, Christiana Care Health Services, Wilmington, Delaware; Department of Family Medicine, and Department of Health Policy, Jefferson Medical College, Philadelphia, Pennsylvania (JMG); and Private Practice, Wilmington, Delaware (AQ)

rheumatic diseases [13,19]. Although there is significant morbidity related to fibromyalgia, there does not seem to be increased mortality. Studies have found no increase in 10-year mortality in fibromyalgia patients [20].

Among adults who seek medical attention for fibromyalgia, less than one third recover within 10 years of onset [21–24]. Symptoms tend to remain stable [22] or improve over time [23,25–27]. Children seem to be much more likely to recover from fibromyalgia, with complete resolution in more than 50% by 2 to 3 years in several studies [3,10,28,29].

DIAGNOSIS OF FIBROMYALGIA AND DIFFUSE MYALGIAS

The most likely cause of chronic diffuse myalgia is fibromyalgia, but other conditions can cause similar symptoms. Before concluding that a patient's symptoms are entirely caused by fibromyalgia, primary care physicians should consider other conditions [6].

Medication-Induced Myalgias

First, the clinician must consider whether diffuse myalgias might be caused by medications. Drug-induced myopathy may occur in persons taking statins, colchicine, corticosteroids, and antimalarial drugs.

Connective Tissues Diseases

Next, connective tissue diseases should be considered. In one study, one fourth of persons referred to a rheumatology clinic with presumed fibromyalgia had a spondyloarthropathy [30]. Dermatomyositis and polymyositis may present with muscle pain and tenderness but, unlike fibromyalgia, cause proximal muscle weakness. Systemic lupus erythematosus, rheumatoid arthritis, and polymyalgia rheumatica can lead to widespread pain. Blood tests, such as an antinuclear antibody (ANA) test, C-reactive protein, or erythrocyte sedimentation rate (ESR), may be helpful in evaluating patients with a history of unexplained rashes, fever, weight loss, joint swelling, iritis, hepatitis, nephritis, or inflammatory back pain (onset before age 40, insidious onset, present for more than 3 months, associated with morning stiffness, improvement with exercise) [31]. In the absence of these signs, anti-nuclear antibody, rheumatoid factor and ESR testing in persons with fatigue and diffuse musculoskeletal pain have low positive predictive value [32]. Rates of false-positive ANAs may be as high as 8% to 11%, especially at low titers [33,34].

Hypothyroidism

Widespread musculoskeletal pain has been associated with hypothyroidism (level of evidence: 3) [35,36], supporting the inclusion of a thyroid-stimulating hormone in the work-up of persons with diffuse myalgias (grade of recommendation: C). More recent research suggests that musculoskeletal pain is more related to thyroid microsomal antibodies than to hypothyroidism [37], but there has been no further evaluation of antithyroid antibodies in persons with diffuse myalgia.

Vitamin D Deficiency and Osteomalacia

Vitamin D deficiency has recently been discovered to be common in the United States, even among persons with lightly pigmented skin [38]. Vitamin D deficiency results in osteomalacia and diffusely aching bones [38]. Persons with fibromyalgia have been found to have high rates of vitamin D deficiency (level of evidence: 3b); therefore, it is reasonable to check these levels in persons with symptoms of fibromyalgia (grade of recommendation: C) [39]. Risk factors include obesity, living at a latitude north of 35 degrees (north of Atlanta and Los Angeles), working indoors year round, advanced age, pigmented skin, and sunblock use [38]. Blood levels of 25-hydroxyvitamin D of <50 ng/mL are considered deficient [38]. Misinterpretation of laboratory results often occurs when clinicians order 1,25-dihydroxyvitamin D levels, which is the active form of the protein found at blood levels that are a thousand-fold less than 25-hydroxyvitamin D. 1,25-dihydroxyvitamin D levels remain normal or elevated in deficient states because increased levels of parathyroid hormone increase renal production of 1,25-dihydroxyvitamin D in response to vitamin D deficiency and decreased intestinal absorption of calcium [38].

DIAGNOSTIC CRITERIA FOR FIBROMYALGIA

The diagnosis of fibromyalgia is based on clinical grounds, as specified in the American College of Rheumatology (ACR) 1990 Criteria for the Classification of Fibromyalgia (Box 1 and Fig. 1) [6]. Fibromyalgia is characterized by widespread pain for at least 3 months, including both sides of the body. The diagnosis of fibromyalgia is based on a combination of the patient's report of widespread pain (right and left sides of the body, above and below the waist, and including the axial skeleton) persisting for at least 3 months and the clinician's identification of at least 11 of 18 potential tender points (level of evidence: 3b) [6].

Despite these well-defined criteria, the diagnosis is not as clear-cut as it may seem to be. The criteria were based on a study of 293 fibromyalgia patients, each of whom had been diagnosed by one of 24 expert investigators according to "his or her usual method of diagnosis" [6]. The investigators identified unique characteristics of fibromyalgia by comparing the 293 cases with 265 control subjects with other chronic pain conditions (low back pain syndromes, neck pain syndromes, regional tendonitis, possible systemic lupus erythematosus, rheumatoid arthritis, or similar disorders). The investigators considered a multitude of symptoms and signs, including sleep disturbance, morning stiffness, paresthesias,

---

Box 1. Clinical Evaluation of Fibromyalgia

IF:

   History: Three months widespread pain defined as pain on the right and left sides of the body (including shoulder and buttock pain) and above and below the waist and including the axial skeleton (cervical spine, anterior chest, thoracic spine, or low back) (grade of recommendation: C)

THEN:

   Physical examination: Complaint of pain rated as 2/10 (0 no pain, 10 worst pain) upon palpation with enough pressure to whiten fingernail in 11 of 18 sites as listed in Fig. 1 (grade of recommendation: C)

THEN:

   Fibromyalgia diagnosed (grade of recommendation: C)

THEN:

   Additional history and examination: Consider other causes of diffuse myalgia, such as medication-induced myalgias, hypothyroidism, osteomalacia, and connective tissue disease (grade of recommendation: D).

THEN:

   Testing: Thyroid-stimulating hormone (grade of recommendation: C), 25-hydroxyvitamin D (grade of recommendation: D), and ESR (grade of recommendation: D), with any additional targeted testing (grade of recommendation: D)

---

irritable bowel syndrome, fatigue, and anxiety, and determined that widespread pain and tender points were the most "sensitive (88.4%) and specific (81.1%)" distinguishing criteria [6]. In this study, calculations of sensitivity and specificity are less meaningful than in studies where an independent reference standard or gold standard is available.

When the 1990 ACR criteria are applied to the general population, there is a continuum of numbers of tender points and pain that is proportionate to overall morbidity; a person with fewer than 11 tender points may experience significant morbidity, suggesting that strict adherence to the ACR criteria may result in many false negatives [40–42]. As suggested by Wolfe in 1997, "the tender point count functions as a sedimentation rate for distress" in persons with chronic pain [42]. The authors of the 1990 ACR study stated that ACR criteria should not be applied rigidly in diagnosing and treating fibromyalgia [42], leaving the diagnosis largely to clinician judgment.

A final difficulty with the diagnostic criteria for fibromyalgia is the dependence on patient report and examiner technique [6]. In the 1990 ACR criteria, tender points were defined as a complaint of pain (or any more dramatic response) upon application of 4 kg of pressure with the pulp of the thumb or first two or three fingers, calibrated using a dolorimeter (a device that can measure the amount and rate of pressure applied over a specified surface area) [6]. It has been shown that practitioners require training to

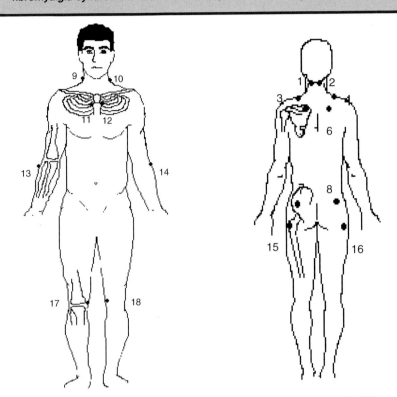

FIGURE 1.
Manual tender point survey. (Adapted from Okifuji A, Turk DC, Sinclair JD, et al. A standardized manual tender point survey: I. development and determination of a threshold point for the identification of positive tender points in fibromyalgia syndrome. J Rheumatol 1997;24:377–83; with permission.)

4 kg pressure is applied at a rate of 1 kg of force per second, using the thumb pad of the dominant hand. Palpate each site only once without probing. The patient is instructed to rate pain after each palpation from 0 (no pain) to 10 (worst pain ever experienced). A rating of 2 or more identifies a tender point.

	R	L
Patient seated		
Occiput: Suboccipital muscle insertions...	1.__	2.__
Trapezius: Midpoint of upper border	3.__	4.__
Supraspinatus: Above scapular spine near medial border	5.__	6.__
Gluteal: Upper outer quadrant of buttocks at anterior edge of gluteus maximus	7.__	8.__
Low cervical: Anterior aspect of the interspaces between the transverse processes of C5-7	9.__	10.__
2nd Rib: Just lateral to 2nd costochondral junction	11.__	12.__
Lateral epicondyle: 2 cm distal to lateral epicondyle	13.__	14.__
Patient on side		
Greater trochanter: 2cm posterior to the greater trochanteric prominence	15.__	16.__
Patient supine		
Knee: Medial fat pad proximal to the joint line	17.__	18.__

apply 4-kg of force with regularity [43]. However, applying exactly 4 kg of pressure may not be clinically important because other studies have demonstrated that the use of finger palpation or dolorimetry identifies tender points with equal accuracy (level of evidence: 3b) [44,45]. Until a more objective test is available, the diagnosis of fibromyalgia will depend mostly on clinical judgment (grade of recommendation: C).

AEROBIC EXERCISE AND OTHER NONPHARMACOLOGIC TREATMENTS

Although aerobic exercise has no significant effect on pain, aerobic exercise exerts other positive effects in persons with fibromyalgia (level of evidence: 1a; grade of recommendation: A). A 2003 Cochrane review identified seven high-quality studies of aerobic training, defined as (1) frequency of 2 days per week; (2) intensity sufficient to achieve 40% to 85% of heart rate reserve or 55% to 90% predicted maximum heart rate; (3) duration of sessions of 20 to 60 minutes duration, continuously or intermittently throughout the day, and using any mode of aerobic exercise; and (4) total time period of at least 6 weeks [46]. Study subjects undertook aerobic dancing, whole body aerobics, stationary cycling, and walking. Subjects who exercised improved in measures of global well being, physical function, aerobic fitness (about 17%), and pain threshold of tender points (about 35%) [46]. In long-term studies, improvements were noted at up to 1 year after treatment ended but not as long as 4.5 years [46]. This Cochrane review strengthens the indication from earlier studies [47,48] that aerobic exercise is beneficial for persons with fibromyalgia.

Other nonpharmacologic treatments for fibromyalgia include educational interventions, relaxation therapy, cognitive-behavioral therapy (CBT), and acupuncture. Although these therapies have been tested in rigorous studies, the heterogeneity of the studies makes it difficult to draw strong conclusions across studies [47]. A systematic review of acupuncture identified only one high-quality RCT showing some improvement in symptoms (grade of recommendation: D) [49].

One therapeutic approach that seems more promising is multidisciplinary rehabilitation. One randomized clinical trial found that combining biofeedback, CBT, exercise, and education resulted in better outcomes than education alone [50]. Other studies have found similar results when combining exercise or CBT with education [51,52]. A meta-analysis concluded that multidisciplinary treatment incorporating physically based and psychologically based treatments was more successful than treatment with a single modality [48]. However, a recent Cochrane review found the evidence on multidisciplinary approaches to be less convincing. The authors concluded that although some physical training plus education had a positive effect at long-term follow-up, current evidence is insufficient to recommend multidisciplinary rehabilitation (grade of recommendation: D) [53].

PHARMACOLOGIC TREATMENT

Of all pharmacologic treatments, antidepressant therapies have undergone the most thorough study. Three meta-analyses have reported that antidepressants, most commonly amitriptyline, improve symptoms for up to several months (level of evidence: 1a; grade of recommendation: A) [54,55]. Pooled results from 13 studies of different antidepressant classes (primarily tricyclics, with three studies of selective serotonin reuptake inhibitors and two of s-adenosylmethionine) revealed a moderate effect on pain, sleep, and global well-being and a mild effect on fatigue and number of trigger points [54]. The authors calculated that persons with fibromyalgia treated with antidepressants were four times more likely to improve than persons treated with placebo. However, they felt that the evidence was much stronger for tricyclic antidepressants than for other antidepressants [54]. Adverse effects seemed to be insignificant but were poorly reported in the individual studies.

A second meta-analysis found that tricyclic antidepressants (generally in doses lower that that used to treat depression) led to improved outcomes; the most improvements were seen in sleep and global assessment, and the least improvements were seen in stiffness and tenderness [55]. The evidence was stronger for tricyclic antidepressants than for other antidepressants. A third meta-analysis of trials using different antidepressants (amitriptyline, dothiepin, fluoxetine, citalopram, and S-adenosyl-methionine) demonstrated improvements in physical status, fibromyalgia symptoms, and psychologic status with no improvement in daily functioning [48].

Another medication that has been found to be beneficial is cyclobenzaprine (level of evidence: 1a; grade of recommendation: A). A recent meta-analysis concluded that cyclobenzaprine was beneficial for patients with fibromyalgia in doses of 10 to 40 mg/d [56] One reason for the benefit of cyclobenzaprine is that, although it is most commonly used as a muscle relaxant, it is structurally similar to the tricyclic antidepressants [57]. Studies have found that the general category of muscle relaxants have no significant benefit [48,55].

The analgesic tramadol has been found to benefit patients with fibromyalgia (level of evidence: 1b; grade of recommendation: A). Several randomized controlled trials showed that the use of tramadol resulted in decreased pain scores [58,59]. This was true when tramadol was used with [58] or without [59] acetaminophen. There is no evidence of benefit for nonsteroidal anti-inflammatory drugs (NSAIDs) [48,55].

In summary, the best evidence supports the use of aerobic exercise and antidepressants in the treatment of fibromyalgia. Regarding antidepressants, the evidence is much stronger for tricyclic antidepressants (particularly amitriptyline and cyclobenzaprine) than for selective serotonin reuptake inhibitors (SSRIs). The only SSRI that has been extensively studied is fluoxetine [57]. The analgesic tramadol also seems to have some benefit in reducing pain, but NSAIDs do not.

Key Points

- Fibromyalgia is common in the general population, effecting up to 2% of adults.
- Fibromyalgia can cause significant morbidity, including higher rates of hospitalization and surgery; however, there is no known relation to mortality.
- Fibromyalgia is diagnosed based on the patient's report of widespread pain of ≥3 months duration and identification of 11 of 18 tender points.
- Before diagnosing fibromyalgia, other causes of diffuse myalgias should be considered, including medications (especially statins), hypothyroidism, osteomalacia, and connective tissue diseases.
- Aerobic exercise improves function and reduces pain in persons with fibromyalgia.
- Antidepressant medications have been shown to moderately improve symptoms in fibromyalgia, although the best evidence is for amitriptyline and other tricyclics.
- Other medications found to be beneficial include cyclobenzaprine and tramadol (with or without acetaminophen).

References

[1] Wolfe F, Ross K, Anderson J, et al. The prevalence and characteristics of fibromyalgia in the general population. Arthritis Rheum 1995;38:19–28.

[2] Buskila D, Press J, Gedalia A, et al. Assessment of nonarticular tenderness and prevalence of fibromyalgia in children. J Rheumatol 1993;20:368–70.

[3] Mikkelsson M. One year outcome of preadolescents with fibromyalgia. J Rheumatol 1999;26:674–82.

[4] Clark P, Burgos-Vargas R, Medina-Palma C, et al. Prevalence of fibromyalgia in children: a clinical study of Mexican children. J Rheumatol 1998;25:2009–14.

[5] White KP, Speechley M, Harth M, et al. The London fibromyalgia epidemiology study: the prevalence of fibromyalgia in London, Ontario. J Rheumatol 1999;26:1570–6.

[6] Wolfe F, Smythe HA, Yunus MB, et al. The American College of Rheumatology 1990 criteria for the classification of fibromyalgia. Arthritis Rheum 1990;33:160–72.

[7] White KP, Speechley M, Harth M, et al. The London fibromyalgia epidemiology study: comparing the demographic and clinical characteristics in 100 random community cases of fibromyalgia versus controls. J Rheumatol 1999;26:1577–85.

[8] Wolfe F, Hawley DJ. Evidence of disordered symptom appraisal in fibromyalgia: increased rates of reported comorbidity and comorbidity severity. Clin Exp Rheumatol 1999;17:297–303.

[9] Leventhal LJ. Management of fibromyalgia. Ann Intern Med 1999;131:850–8.

[10] Gedalia A, Garcia CO, Molina JF, et al. Fibromyalgia syndrome: experience in a pediatric rheumatology clinic. Clin Exp Rheumatol 2000;18:415–9.

[11] Yunus MB, Masi AT. Juvenile primary fibromyalgia syndrome: a clinical study of thirty-three patients and matched normal controls. Arthritis Rheum 1985;28:138–45.

[12] Tayag-Kier CE, Keenan GF, Scalzi LV, et al. Sleep and periodic limb movement in sleep in juvenile fibromyalgia. Pediatrics 2000;106:E70.

[13] Wolfe F, Anderson J, Harkness D, et al. A prospective longitudinal, multicenter study of service utilization and costs in fibromyalgia. Arthritis Rheum 1997;40:1560–70.

[14] Jason LA, Taylor RR, Kennedy CL. Chronic fatigue. Psychosom Med 2000;62:655–63.

[15] Hedenberg-Magnusson B, Ernberg M, Kopp S. Presence of orofacial pain and temporomandibular disorder in fibromyalgia: a study by questionnaire. Swed Dent J 1999;23:185–92.

[16] Henriksson C, Liedberg G. Factors of importance for work disability in women with fibromyalgia. J Rheumatol 2000;27:1271–6.

[17] White KP, Speechley M, Harth M, et al. Comparing self-reported function and work disability in 100 community cases of fibromyalgia syndrome versus controls in London, Ontario: the London fibromyalgia epidemiology study. Arthritis Rheum 1999;42:76–83.

[18] Swezey RL, Adams J. Fibromyalgia: a risk factor for osteoporosis. J Rheumatol 1999;26: 2642–4.

[19] ter Borg EJ, Gerards-Rociu E, Haanen HC, et al. High frequency of hysterectomies and appendectomies in fibromyalgia compared with rheumatoid arthritis: a pilot study. Clin Rheumatol 1999;18:1–3.

[20] Makela M, Heliovaara M. Prevalence of primary fibromyalgia in the Finnish population. BMJ 1991;303:216–9.

[21] Forseth KO, Forre O, Gran JT. A 5.5 year prospective study of self-reported musculoskeletal pain and of fibromyalgia in a female population: significance and natural history. Clin Rheumatol 1999;18:114–21.

[22] Wolfe F, Anderson J, Harkness D, et al. Health status and disease severity in fibromyalgia: results of a six-center longitudinal study. Arthritis Rheum 1997;40:1571–9.

[23] Kennedy M, Felson DT. A prospective long-term study of fibromyalgia syndrome. Arthritis Rheum 1996;39:682–5.

[24] Waylonis GW, Perkins RH. Post-traumatic fibromyalgia. a long-term follow-up. Am J Phys Med Rehabil 1994;73:403–12.

[25] Baumgartner E, Finckh A, Cedraschi C, et al. A six year prospective study of a cohort of patients with fibromyalgia. Ann Rheum Dis 2002;61:644–5.

[26] Mengshoel AM, Haugen M. Health status in fibromyalgia-a followup study. J Rheumatol 2001;28:2085–9.

[27] Poyhia R, DaCosta D, Fitzcharles MA. Pain and pain relief in fibromyalgia patients followed for three years. Arthritis Rheum 2001;45:355–61.

[28] Buskila D, Neumann L, Hershman E, et al. Fibromyalgia syndrome in children: an outcome study. J Rheumatol 1995;22:525–8.

[29] Siegel DM, Janeway D, Baum J. Fibromyalgia syndrome in children and adolescents: clinical features at presentation and status at follow-up. Pediatrics 1998;101:377–82.

[30] Fitzcharles MA, Esdaile JM. The overdiagnosis of fibromyalgia syndrome. Am J Med 1997;103:44–50.

[31] Dougados M, van der Linden S, Juhlin R, et al. The European Spondylarthropathy Study Group preliminary criteria for the classification of spondylarthropathy. Arthritis Rheum 1991;34:1218–27.

[32] Suarez-Almazor ME, Gonzalez-Lopez L, Gamez-Nava JI, et al. Utilization and predictive value of laboratory tests in patients referred to rheumatologists by primary care physicians. J Rheumatol 1998;25:1980–5.

[33] Al-Allaf AW, Ottewell L, Pullar T. The prevalence and significance of positive antinuclear antibodies in patients with fibromyalgia syndrome: 2–4 years' follow-up. Clin Rheumatol 2002;21:472–7.

[34] Yunus MB, Hussey FX, Aldag JC. Antinuclear antibodies and connective tissue disease features in fibromyalgia syndrome: a controlled study. J Rheumatol 1993;20: 1557–60.

[35] Carette S, Lefrancois L. Fibrositis and primary hypothyroidism. J Rheumatol 1988;15: 1418–21.

[36] Delamere JP, Scott DL, Felix-Davies DD. Thyroid dysfunction and rheumatic diseases. J R Soc Med 1982;75:102–6.

[37] Aarflot T, Bruusgaard D. Association between chronic widespread musculoskeletal complaints and thyroid autoimmunity: results from a community survey. Scand J Prim Health Care 1996;14:111–5.

[38] Holick MF. Vitamin D: importance in the prevention of cancers, type 1 diabetes, heart disease, and osteoporosis [erratum appears in Am J Clin Nutr 2004;79:890] Am J Clin Nutr 2004;79:362–71.

[39] Al-Allaf AW, Mole PA, Paterson CR, et al. Bone health in patients with fibromyalgia. Rheumatology 2002;42:1202–6.

[40] Croft P, Schollum J, Silman A. Population study of tender point counts and pain as evidence of fibromyalgia. BMJ 1994;309:696–9.

[41] Croft P, Burt J, Schollum J, et al. More pain, more tender points: is fibromyalgia just one end of a continuous spectrum? Ann Rheum Dis 1996;55:482–5.

[42] Wolfe F. The relation between tender points and fibrymyalgia symptom variables: evidence that fibromyalgia is not a discrete disorder in the clinic. Ann Rheum Dis 1997;56:268–71.

[43] Smythe H. Examination for tenderness: learning to use 4 kg force. J Rheumatol 1998;25: 149–51.

[44] Tunks E, McCain GA, Hart LE, et al. The reliability of examination for tenderness in patients with myofacial pain, chronic fibromyalgia and controls. J Rheumatol 1995;22: 944–52.

[45] Jacobs JW, Geenen R, van der Heide A, et al. Are tender point scores assessed by manual palpation in fibromyalgia reliable? An investigation into the variance of tender point scores. Scand J Rheumatol 1995;24:243–7.

[46] Busch A, Schachter CL, Peloso PM, et al. Exercise for treating fibromyalgia syndrome. Cochrane Database Syst Rev 2002;3:CD003786.

[47] Sim J, Adams N. Systematic review of randomized controlled trials of nonpharmacological interventions for fibromyalgia. Clin J Pain 2002;18:324–36.

[48] Rossy LA, Buckelew SP, Dorr N, et al. A meta-analysis of fibromyalgia treatment interventions. Ann Behav Med 1999;21:180–91.

[49] Berman BM, Ezzo J, Hadhazy V, et al. Is acupuncture effective in the treatment of fibromyalgia? J Fam Pract 1999;48:213–8.

[50] Buckelew SP, Conway R, Parker J, et al. Biofeedback/relaxation training and exercise interventions for fibromyalgia: a prospective trial. Arthritis Care Res 1998;11:196–209.

[51] Keel PJ, Bodoky C, Gerhard U, et al. Comparison of integrated group therapy and group relaxation training for fibromyalgia. Clin J Pain 1998;14:232–8.

[52] King SJ, Wessel J, Bhambhani Y, et al. The effects of exercise and education, individually or combined, in women with fibromyalgia. J Rheumatol 2002;29:2620–7.

[53] Karjalainen K, Malmivaara A, van Tulder M, et al. Multidisciplinary rehabilitation for fibromyalgia and musculoskeletal pain in working age adults. Cochrane Database Syst Rev 2000;2:CD001984.

[54] O'Malley PG, Balden E, Tomkins G, et al. Treatment of fibromyalgia with antidepressants: a meta-analysis. J Gen Itern Med 2000;15:659–66.

[55] Arnold LM, Keck PE, Welge JA. Antidepressment treatment of fibromyalgia: a meta-analysis and review. Psychosomatics 2000;41:104–13.

[56] Tofferi JK, Jackson JL, O'Malley PG. Treatment of fibromyalgia with cyclobenzaprine: a meta-analysis. Arthritis Rheum 2004;51:9–13.

[57] Goldenberg DL, Burckhardt C, Crofford L. Management of fibromyalgia syndrome. JAMA 2004;292:2388–95.

[58] Bennett RM, Kamin M, Karim R, et al. Tramadol and acetaminophen combination tablets in the treatment of fibromyalgia pain: a double-blind, randomized, placebo-controlled study. Am J Med 2003;114:537–45.

[59] Russell J, Kamin M, Bennet R, et al. Efficacy of tramadol in treatment of pain in fibromyalgia. J Clin Rheumatol 2000;6:250–7.

Address reprint requests to

James M. Gill, MD, MPH
Department of Family and Community Medicine
1401 Foulk Road
Wilmington, DE 19803

e-mail: jgill@christianacare.org

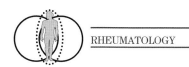
LYME DISEASE

Andrew J. Foy, Jr., BS, and James Studdiford, MD, FACP

Lyme disease (LD) is a systemic illness resulting from infection with the spirochete *Borrelia burgdorferi* [1]. Based on the Centers for Disease Control and Prevention (CDC) definition for reportable cases of LD, the number of cases increased from 7943 cases in 1990 to 17,730 cases in 2000 [2,3]. The highest prevalence of LD occurs in children 2 to 15 years of age and in persons 30 to 59 years of age [3]. In 2000, 48 out of 50 states reported cases of LD, with the highest prevalence being reported in the mid-Atlantic region and along the northeast corridor of the United States [2]. (Fig. 1) shows the endemicity of LD in a particular area of the country.

LD is associated with a variety of signs and symptoms that may present at different stages of infection. The stages include early localized, early disseminated, and late chronic (Table 1). The onset of clinical manifestations of LD typically occurs between 7 and 10 days after a tick bite, with a reported range of 1 to 36 days [4]. Most patients (60% to 80%) develop the early, localized form of LD characterized by erythema migrans (EM) and flu-like symptoms [5].

Research suggests that EM most commonly presents as a slowly expanding erythematous lesion with central clearing in the shape of a bull's eye (Fig. 2) [6]. A recent observational cohort study reported that 50% of EM lesions in a highly endemic area were homogeneous, with 34% showing central redness (Fig. 3) [7]. A punctum from the original tick bite was present 30% of the time (Fig. 4) [7]. The erythematous lesion with partial central clearing, formerly thought to be classic for LD, was found in only 9% of cases (Fig. 5) [7].

Early LD without EM was once thought to be a rare finding, and some experts believed that these patients were more likely to have human granulocytic ehrlichiosis (HGE) or babesiosis than LD [8]; however, a recent study found that in endemic areas during the summer months, 18% of individuals with LD presented with constitutional symptoms without EM [9]. Their most common symptoms were headache and arthralgia, sometimes associated with fever [9].

From Jefferson Medical College, Philadelphia, Pennsylvania

FIGURE 1.
Map of endemicity for Lyme Disease.

National Lyme disease risk map with four categories of risk

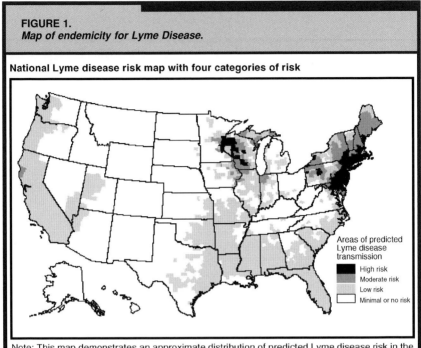

Areas of predicted
Lyme disease
transmission

■ High risk
▨ Moderate risk
▒ Low risk
☐ Minimal or no risk

Note: This map demonstrates an approximate distribution of predicted Lyme disease risk in the United States. The true relative risk in any given county compared with other counties might differ from that shown here and might change from year to year. Risk categories are defined in the accompanying text. Information on risk distribution within states and counties is best obtained from state and local public health authorities.

Early disseminated LD affects the nervous system, heart, and joints with clinical manifestations evolving over weeks to months in a relatively painless fashion [10]. The most common acute neurologic abnormalities are seventh nerve palsy, meningitis, and radiculoneuropathy, which alone or in combination affect 15% of untreated patients [10]. Lyme carditis classically involves the conduction system, with sudden occurrence of high-grade atrioventricular block resulting in palpitations, light-headedness, and syncope [10]. The typical acute arthritic attack of early disseminated LD varies considerably from that of late LD and is generally characterized as monoarticular with only one knee being affected [10]. Sudden pain and swelling with massive effusions (Fig. 6) are common, and most patients experience intermittent attacks [10].

Late LD is generally confined to the nervous system and joints. The term describes the continuous inflammation in a specific organ system for more than 1 year. Late Lyme arthritis is characterized by persistent inflammatory arthritis of one or two large joints, most often the knee [10]. The histologic lesion of late Lyme arthritis mimics that of rheumatoid arthritis; this differs considerably from the lesion of early disseminated Lyme arthritis [10]. The best described manifestations of late neurologic

TABLE 1.
Clinical Features of Lyme Disease

System	Stage 1 (Early) Localized	Stage 2 (Early) Disseminated	Stage 3 (Late) Chronic
Skin	Erythema migrans	Secondary annular lesions	
Musculoskeletal	Myalgia, arthralgia	Migratory pain in joints; brief arthritis attacks	Prolonged arthritis attacks, chronic arthritis
Neurologic	Headache	Meningitis, Bell palsy, cranial neuritis, radiculoneuritis	Encephalopathy, polyneuropathy, leukoencephalitis
Cardiac		Atrioventricular block, myopericarditis, pancarditis	
Constitutional	Flu-like symptoms	Malaise, fatigue	Fatigue
Lymphatic	Regional lymphadenopathy	Regional or generalized lymphadenopathy	

LD are a subtle sensory-radiculoneuropathy and a low-grade encephalopathy presenting with deficits in cognitive function affecting concentration, learning, and short-term memory [10].

Clinical manifestations of LD in children resemble those in adults. The most common clinical manifestation of LD in children is the EM rash followed by arthritis, facial nerve palsy, aseptic meningitis, and carditis [3]. Lyme meningitis has been reported in children with facial nerve palsy [11]. As in adults, Lyme meningitis in children may be subtle and usually occurs

FIGURE 2.
Bull's eye rash.

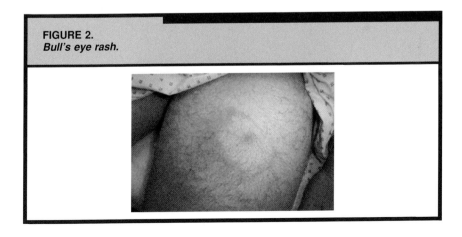

FIGURE 3.
Erythema migrans with central redness.

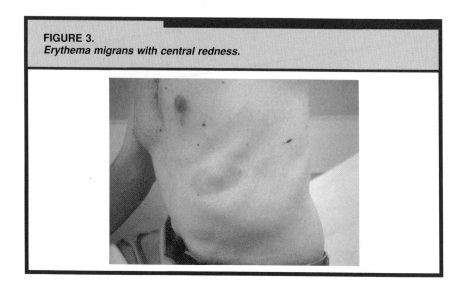

without meningismus. When compared with children with viral meningitis, children with Lyme meningitis presented with significantly less fever but similar rates of headache, neck pain, and malaise [12].

Coinfection of patients with other tick-borne illnesses, such as *Babesia microti* and rickettsial-like pathogens causing HGE, has been

FIGURE 4.
Homogeneous erythema migrans with central punctum.

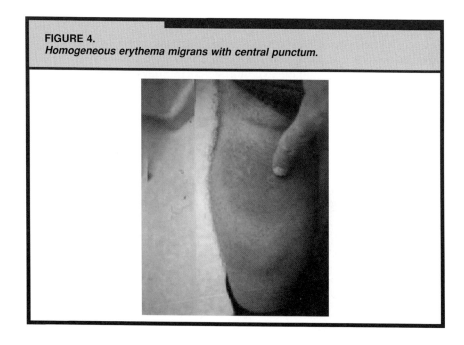

FIGURE 5.
Erythematous lesion with partial central clearing.

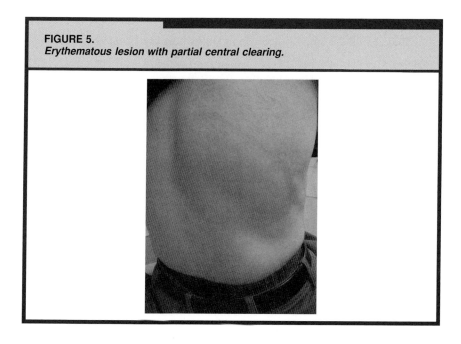

reported [13,14]. Coinfected patients commonly present with a prolonged flu-like illness, often highlighted by thrombocytopenia [13,14].

The most widely accepted guidelines for the diagnosis of LD are from the American College of Physicians (ACP), who used the 1990 CDC surveillance criteria (outlined in Box 1). Due to the limitations of

FIGURE 6.
Knee effusion in early disseminated Lyme Disease.

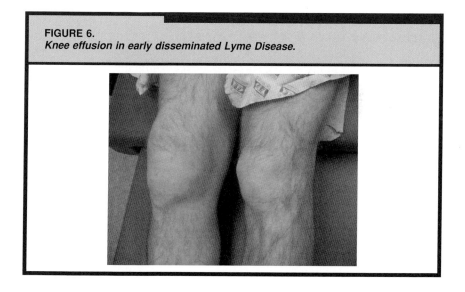

Box 1. CDC 1990 Clinical Case Definition for Lyme Disease

Clinical Case Definition: (1) Erythema migrans or (2) at least one advanced manifestation as defined below, and laboratory confirmation of infection.

Advanced Manifestations
- *Musculoskeletal system*—Recurrent brief attacks lasting weeks or months of objective joint swelling in one or a few joints, sometimes followed by chronic arthritis in one or a few joints. Manifestations not considered criteria for diagnosis include chronic progressive arthritis not preceded by brief attacks and chronic symmetrical polyarthritis. Arthralgia, myalgia, or fibromyalgia syndromes alone are not criteria for musculoskeletal involvement.
- *Nervous system*—Any of the following, alone or in combination: lymphocytic meningitis; cranial neuritis, particularly facial palsy (may be bilateral); radiculoneuropathy; or rarely encephalomyelitis (must be confirmed by showing antibody production against B burgdorferi in the CSF, demonstrated by a higher titer of antibody in CSF than in serum). Headache, fatigue, paresthesia, and mild stiff neck alone are not criteria for neurologic involvement.
- *Cardiovascular system*—Acute-onset, high-grade (2 or 3) atrioventricular conduction defects that resolve in days to weeks and are sometimes associated with myocarditis. Palpitations, bradycardia, bundle-branch block, or myocarditis are not criteria for cardiovascular involvement.

Adapted from MMWR 1990;9:1–43.

---

laboratory testing for LD, diagnosis is based primarily on clinical findings, such as EM rash [5,7,16,17]. Specific serologic tests should be used to confirm a clinical diagnosis of LD only when patients present with a moderate to low pretest probability of having the disease.

LABORATORY TESTS FOR LYME DISEASE

The host antibody response to *B burgdorferi* infection develops slowly, and only about half of patients with early-stage LD have a positive serology. The IgM and IgG antibodies appear 2 to 4 and 4 to 6 weeks, respectively, after the onset of EM and peak at 6 to 8 weeks [17]. Although IgM may persist indefinitely, it usually declines to low levels after 4 to 6 months of illness, whereas IgG remains present at low but significant levels despite successful treatment [17]. Therefore, the physician must evaluate the significance of a serologic result in the context of the patient's epidemiologic history.

Serologic testing provides poor results for patients presenting with EM rash because of the difference in time that it takes for EM to appear (7 to 10 days) versus the time it takes for IgM and IgG antibodies to appear (2 to 4 and 4 to 6 weeks, respectively). Serologic testing may provide valuable information in two distinct sets of patients: (1) patients with endemic exposure and clinical findings that suggest later-stage disseminated LD or

(2) patients with prolonged constitutional symptoms (≥ 2 weeks) that may suggest the early stages of LD in the absence of EM. Early diagnosis is crucial in group 2 because untreated infection can result in advanced disease involving the nervous system or joints, which is less responsive to treatment [15].

When serologic testing is indicated, one should use the two-step approach recommended by the CDC-ASTPHLD (Center for Disease Control – Association of State and Territorial Public Health Laboratory Directors), in which a positive or indeterminate ELISA is followed by a more specific Western blot (grade of recommendation: A) [18]. Positive ELISA samples drawn from patients within 4 weeks of disease onset should undergo Western blotting for IgM and IgG. Samples drawn more than 4 weeks from disease onset are tested for IgG only [18]. Most commercial labs empirically test for IgM and IgG regardless of the reported time from disease onset; therefore, clinicians must look only at the IgG results if samples were drawn more than 4 weeks after onset because the risk of false positives with IgM at this late stage is high [18]. In summary, for a patient with serum drawn more than 4 weeks after the onset of symptoms, a positive IgM result with a negative IgG should be looked at as a false positive; however, if IgM and IgG or just IgG are positive, then it should be viewed as a true positive.

The specificity of this two-step approach in early or late stage disease is 95% to 100%, compared with 80% for serology alone, decreasing the number of false-positive results [18,19]. Table 2 shows the accuracy of individual tests and the combined two-step approach. When ordering laboratory tests for LD, clinicians should report the time in weeks from the onset of disease.

DIAGNOSIS

A critical factor in the interpretation of laboratory tests for LD is the pretest probability of disease. This is the physician's estimate of the likelihood of LD given the geographic location and the patient's signs and symptoms. If the pretest probability is high, a negative test is more likely to be a false negative. Conversely, if the pretest probability is low, a positive test is more likely to be a false positive. Fig. 1 and Table 3 provide guidance on estimating the pretest probability in LD cases.

ACP recommendations suggest that the diagnosis of early LD can be made on clinical grounds alone when the pretest probability is high (>80%). This includes individuals who reside in an area of high endemicity who have EM rash. These patients should be diagnosed and treated without testing (grade of recommendation: A).

Individuals who reside in areas of moderate endemicity and present with EM rash have not been previously categorized into the high or moderate pretest probability groups. In addition, it has been difficult to identify research from moderately endemic areas to suggest the percentage of patients presenting with erythematous lesions who have

TABLE 2.
Accuracy of Diagnostic Tests for Lyme Disease

Diagnostic Test and Stage of LD	Sensitivity, %	Specificity, %	LR+	LR−	Probability of LD for Positive Tests Given Different Pretest Probabilities		
					2%	10%	50%
Serology (alone) in early-stage disease [7]	59	93	8.4	0.44	13–15	46–49	86–89
Serology (alone) in late-stage disease [7]	95	81	5.0	0.06	10	38–39	81–82
Serology + Western blot in early and late stages[a] [15,16]	50–75[b]	99–100	50–75	0.4–0.5	50–55	85–87	97–98

Abbreviation: LD, Lyme disease.
[a] Only studies were included that followed the complete criteria for two-step testing following the CDC-ASTPHLD guidelines in which samples that were positive or equivocal for serology, drawn within 4 weeks of disease onset, were followed by IgG and IgM Western blots and in which samples drawn after 4 weeks of disease onset were followed only by IgG Western blots.
[b] Decrease in sensitivity is associated with a lack of antibody response or seroconversion in patients treated with LD with antibiotics.

TABLE 3.
Estimating Pretest Probability and Using it to Guide Interpretation of Serologic Testing

Endemicity of LD[a]	Objective Clinical Signs and Symptoms	Pretest Probability	Laboratory Testing
High, moderate, or low	Absent	Very low (eg, <5%)	Not recommended (high false-positive rate)
Low	Absent, but has prolonged, unexplained nonspecific symptoms	Very low	Not recommended
Moderate/high	Absent, but has prolonged, unexplained nonspecific symptoms	Moderately low (eg, ≤5% to 20%)	Should be considered
Moderate	Present (without EM)	Moderate (eg, 20% to 80%)	Recommended
Moderate/low	EM present	Moderate–high	Not recommended (high false-negative rate); diagnosis of LD based on clinical grounds alone should be considered
High	EM present	High (eg, ≥80%)	Not recommended (high false-negative rate); diagnose LD based on clinical grounds alone

Abbreviations: EM, erythema migrans; LD, Lyme disease.
[a] See Fig. 1.

LD. Therefore, we suggest that these patients be treated empirically if the clinician can be reasonably certain the rash is an EM rash (grade of recommendation: D). In these cases, clinicians should take a detailed history, taking into account the patient's risk of exposure and the presence or absence of flu-like symptoms, which if present are generally a good indicator of LD.

Individuals residing in areas of high or moderate endemicity who present with objective signs and symptoms of LD (see Box 1) in the absence of EM rash have an intermediate probability of LD (20% to 80%). These patients should have two-step testing (ELISA followed by confirmatory Western blot) with treatment guided by the results (grade of recommendation: A).

When the pretest probability of LD is low (<20%), serologic testing is controversial. This group includes individuals who present with only nonspecific, constitutional symptoms of LD (eg, flu-like symptoms, arthralgia, myalgia, paresthesia, etc.) or asymptomatic patients who present with a request for screening. The ACP guidelines recommend that physicians minimize laboratory testing in these individuals, although other experts have noted the value of the two-step approach in otherwise low-risk individuals from highly endemic areas who have experienced nonspecific symptoms for a sustained period of time [5,15–17]. A recent study found that these patients represent about 18% of LD cases in endemic areas during the summer months [9].

Because patients with early LD without EM make up such a large population of LD patients, it is the author's opinion that they should be tested for LD (grade of recommendation: D). Therefore, it is recommended that individuals from endemic areas with persistent, unexplained constitutional symptoms for ≥2 weeks be tested for LD using the complete two-step approach (grade of recommendation: D). When the CDC-ASTPHLD guidelines are applied to two-step testing, the likelihood that a positive test result indicates true infection is estimated to be 85% to 87%. Two weeks is the recommended cut-off point to initiate two-step testing because of the time it takes for seroconversion to occur. Physicians should be aware that false-negative results can occur due to lack of seroconversion at this early stage of disease.

THE LOW-RISK PATIENT

Three sample clinical scenarios have been devised to help clinicians determine if the two-step approach should be used for individuals with a low pretest probability of LD.

Clinical Scenario A

An individual from an area of high endemicity of LD presents in the spring or summer with several weeks of flu-like symptoms including fever, headache, and arthralgias but no EM rash. After a thorough clinical evaluation, the cause of the symptoms is unresolved.

Approach to Patient A

The clinician in this case should consider serologic testing using the two-step approach. For this individual, the pretest probability is moderately low, taking into account endemicity of disease and the presence of prolonged, unexplained constitutional symptoms of LD. In this scenario, the probability of LD is about 90% if the two-step approach is positive. Although testing and treatment is probably beneficial in these patients, this has not been proven.

Clinical Scenario B

An individual from an area of moderate or high endemicity of LD presents with headache and fatigue but no EM. The symptoms have lasted for 3 days.

Approach to Patient B

The clinician should not order serologic testing because there is a high risk of false positives at this early stage of nonspecific disease (over 50%). The clinician should advise the patient to follow up if symptoms persist. In this scenario, the pretest probability is estimated to be very low.

Clinical Scenario C

A healthy child from a highly endemic area receives an annual physical. The mother requests LD screening tests, noting that the child spends a lot of time playing in the backyard, which is adjacent to a heavily wooded area and that the child's best friend was just diagnosed with LD.

Approach to Patient C

The clinician should not order serologic testing because the child is asymptomatic. A false-positive result would expose the child unnecessarily to the risks of treatment. In this scenario, the probability that a positive test represents true infection is less than 25%.

LIKELY REASONS FOR OBTAINING FALSE-POSITIVE AND FALSE-NEGATIVE TEST RESULTS

A likely reason for obtaining false-positive results is the persistence of IgM and IgG antibody activity, due to previous exposure, in the absence of ongoing infection. A positive result from ELISA alone occurs in about 2% to 5% of healthy individuals living in a region of low endemicity [5,16,17]. As the endemicity of LD increases, so does the rate of positive ELISA results in healthy individuals due to the increased risk of past exposure.

When LD is among the likely differential diagnoses, the most common reason for a positive serology test in the absence of LD is the presence of another spirochetal infection (eg, syphilis), spirochete periodontal infections, or relapsing fever [16]. Patients with rheumatic diseases or with infectious mononucleosis may also have false-positive reactions, especially with IgM [5,15–17].

A high rate of false-positive tests is associated with the withdrawn LYMErix vaccine, which was a recombinant form of the OspA lipoprotein of *B burgdorferi*. Because standard whole-cell kits use in vitro cultivated spirochetes, OspA is one of the antigens present. Therefore, a vaccine will most likely show a positive result in any of the standard whole-cell ELISA kits. To alleviate this problem, physicians should consider ordering only a Western blot and disregarding the OspA band when determining whether the test is positive or negative in vaccinated individuals.

False-negative results are often attributable to tests taken too early in the course of infections. Because the antibody response develops slowly, tests taken within the first 2 weeks of infection have sensitivities less than 50%. Antibiotics can also influence the results of serologic tests when given early in the course of infection and have been shown to abort seroconversion, even if inadequate therapy is given [15]. True seronegativity in the later stages of LD is uncommon [15,16].

PROBLEMS WITH OVERDIAGNOSIS AND MISDIAGNOSIS

Overdiagnosis is most commonly attributable to the incorrect interpretation of Western blot results, misidentification of rashes as EM, and ascribing nonspecific symptoms to LD [20–22]. Western blot results cannot be intermediate and should be classified as negative or positive according to the CDC-ASTPHLD guidelines.

Underdiagnosis may occur if physicians apply the CDC surveillance criteria too strictly (see Box 1), which is meant to be used for research purposes only and not as a diagnostic tool. A recent study showed that patients with prolonged nonspecific symptoms but no EM rash or advanced manifestations of LD make up almost 20% of LD cases in endemic areas during the summer months [9]. All these patients would be missed according to the CDC surveillance criteria.

TREATMENT

Early Lyme Disease: Acute or Disseminated

Treatment for LD should be tailored to the stage of the disease and the age of the patient (Table 4). Patients with early acute or early disseminated LD should be treated with a 10- to 21-day course of first-line antibiotics. Doxycycline (100 mg two times per day), amoxicillin (500 mg three times per day), and cefuroxime axetil (500 mg two times per day) have been proven efficacious for the treatment of early LD [23–28].

Almost all patients with early LD respond promptly and completely to these first-line antibiotics, and objective evidence of treatment failure is uncommon [8]. Subjective symptoms occur in a low percentage of patients after antibiotic therapy and usually remit spontaneously without additional antibiotic therapy.

One study has shown that a 10-day course of doxycycline therapy is as effective as a 20-day course for the treatment of EM and that the addition of a dose of ceftriaxone in the beginning of a 10-day course of doxycycline did not increase efficacy [29]. The same study showed that oral doxycycline was as effective as parenteral ceftriaxone in the treatment of early-stage

TABLE 4.
Treatment of Lyme Disease

Stage	Therapy
Early acute LD	10-day course of oral doxycycline or other oral antibiotics including amoxicillin or cefuroxime axetil if doxycycline contraindicated (grade of recommendation: A)
Early LD without EM	10-day course of oral doxycycline should be considered (grade of recommendation: D)
Early disseminated LD	14- to 21-day course of oral doxycycline or parenteral antibiotics if doxycycline is contraindicated (grade of recommendation: B)
Late Lyme arthritis	Oral or parenteral antibiotic therapies indicated (grade of recommendation: B)
Late LD with neurologic manifestations	Parenteral ceftriaxone recommended (grade of recommendation: C)
Post-LD syndrome	Antibiotic treatment not recommended (grade of recommendation: A)

Abbreviations: EM, erythema migrans; LD, Lyme disease.

LD [7]. Doxycycline is the only antibiotic effective against early LD that is also effective against HGE, which may coexist with LD. One study evaluating the in vitro antibiotic susceptibility of HGE confirmed the observed clinical efficacy and bactericidal activity of doxycycline against HGE [30]. The same study showed that HGE was resistant to ampicillin, ceftriaxone, and other antibiotics commonly used to treat LD [30]. Therefore, patients with early acute LD should be treated with a 10-day course of doxycycline; other first-line antibiotics, such as amoxicillin or cefuroxime axetil, should be used when doxycycline is contraindicated (grade of recommendation: A).

It has been traditionally perceived that oral antibiotics are not effective in treating early disseminated neurologic LD (neuroborreliosis); however, recent studies in adults provide evidence that oral doxycycline is an effective alternative to parenteral antibiotic therapy [31–33]. In a randomized trial of 54 patients with neuroborreliosis, Karlsson et al [33] compared the efficacy of oral doxycycline (200 mg per day for 14 days) to IV penicillin G (3 g every 6 hours for 14 days). Patients in both groups improved during treatment, and there were no significant differences between the two treatment groups in patient scoring, CSF analysis, or serologic and clinical follow-up during 1 year. Dotevall and Hagberg [32] reported a case series of 29 patients with neuroborreliosis, nerve palsy, and meningitis who were treated with oral doxycycline (200 to 400 mg per day for 9 to 17 days). Twenty-six patients (90%) recovered without sequelae within 6 months. The authors recommend that patients with early disseminated neurologic LD be treated with a 14- to 21-day course of oral or parenteral antibiotics if doxycycline is contraindicated (grade of recommendation: B).

Macrolides and first-generation cephalosporins should not be used in the treatment of LD. There is no evidence supporting their effectiveness. One single-blind, randomized study evaluating the macrolide roxithromycin versus penicillin had to be stopped after 19 patients had enrolled due to five treatment failures [34]. In the roxithromycin group, three patients had persisting or recurrent EM, one developed a secondary EM-like lesion and severe arthralgia, and one developed neuroborreliosis. Another study evaluating the outcomes of patients treated with the cephalosporin cephalexin found that 11 out of 11 patients had clinical evidence of disease progression [35]. These manifestations included eight patients whose rash enlarged, two who developed seventh-nerve palsy, and one who developed disseminated EM lesions.

Treatment for early LD should be considered for patients from endemic areas who present with prolonged, unexplained constitutional symptoms in the absence of EM and who test positive for LD (grade of recommendation: C). Approximately 20% of LD can present in this fashion [9]. There is not much evidence to support or dispute that antibiotic treatment of these patients is effective in preventing the progression to late LD. However, one recent study evaluated antibiotic treatment of patients with early LD without EM and reported that late manifestations of LD did not develop in any patient and that subjective symptoms remained in only 11% to 16% of patients treated with antibiotics [9]. These results must be viewed cautiously because there was no control group, and therefore disease progression cannot be conclusively linked to antibiotic therapy.

Late Lyme Disease

Treatment of late LD should be directed to the specific organ system that is involved. Oral and parenteral antibiotic therapies have proven to be effective in treating Lyme arthritis [36–40]. Lack of response to antibiotic therapy has been associated with the combination of HLA-DR4 specificity and OspA or OspB reactivity [38].

Eichenfield et al [37] studied 25 children, aged 2 to 15 years, with Lyme arthritis and reported that antibiotic therapy was effective in all patients and that in 13 of 14 patients, orally administered therapy alone resulted in elimination of synovitis and recurrent attacks. One study randomly assigned patients with persistent Lyme arthritis to receive doxycycline or amoxicillin plus probenecid for 30 days [38]. Eighteen of 20 patients treated with doxycycline and 16 of 18 patients treated with amoxicillin had resolution of the arthritis within 1 to 3 months after study entry. Neuroborreliosis later developed in five patients, four of whom received the amoxicillin regimen.

One double-blind, placebo-controlled trial of 40 patients with established Lyme arthritis found that 7 of 20 patients receiving parenteral penicillin therapy had complete resolution of arthritis soon after injection and remained well during a mean follow-up period of 33 months, whereas all 20 patients given placebo continued to have attacks of arthritis [36]. A similar study found that 11 of 20 patients treated with intravenous penicillin had complete resolution of arthritis [36]. Penicillin-responsive patients in both studies were more likely to have previously received antibiotics for EM and were less likely to have been given intra-articular corticosteroids during or at the conclusion of parenteral therapy [36].

For patients with refractory, chronic arthritis of the knee that persists after treatment with oral and parenteral antibiotic therapy, arthroscopic synovectomy is an effective treatment option (grade of recommendation: C). Schoen et al [39] reported that 16 of 20 patients who underwent arthroscopic synovectomy for refractory chronic Lyme arthritis had resolution of joint inflammation during the first month after surgery or soon thereafter and remained well during the 3- to 8-year follow-up period.

Parenteral therapy is indicated for patients suffering from late neuroborreliosis (grade of recommendation: C). Ceftriaxone is the best-studied antibiotic for treatment of patients with neurologic symptoms associated with late LD [40,41]. In a case series of 18 patients with Lyme encephalopathy that developed months to years after classic manifestations of LD, Logician et al [40] reported that 16 (89%) had abnormal memory scores, and seven out of seven patients tested with SPECT imaging had frontotemporal perfusion defects. All patients were treated with an intravenous ceftriaxone regimen of 2 g per day for 30 days. Six months after treatment, memory scores in the 15 patients who completed the study according to protocol were significantly improved. Twelve to 24 months after treatment, all 18 patients rated themselves as back to normal or improved.

Post-Lyme Disease Syndrome

There is no evidence to support the use of antibiotics to treat post-Lyme disease syndrome. Several double-blind, randomized, placebo-controlled trials have shown that providing additional antibiotic therapy to seropositive and seronegative patients with post-Lyme disease syndrome is not more beneficial than administering placebo [42,43]. It has been recommended that physicians do not treat these individuals with antibiotics but instead treat the symptoms and look for other causes to explain them (grade of recommendation: A).

One randomized study evaluated whether prolonged antibiotic treatment was effective for patients with persistent musculoskeletal pain, neurocognitive symptoms, or dysesthesia often associated with fatigue after the recommended antibiotic treatment for acute LD [42]. Seventy-eight patients who were seropositive and 51 patients who were sero-negative for IgG antibodies to *B burgdorferi* were studied. Among seropositive patients treated with prolonged antibiotics, there was improvement in the score on the physical component summary scale of the SF-36, the mental component summary scale, or both in 37%; there was no change in 29%, and there was worsening in 34%. Among seropositive patients who received placebo, there was improvement in 40%, no change in 26%, and worsening in 34%; the results were similar for the seronegative patients.

Key Points

- When considering the diagnosis of lyme disease, the physician must take into account the patient's pretest probability of having the disease.
- Individuals with erythema migrans should not be tested for lyme disease (LD). Instead, the physician can make the diagnosis based on the patient's history and the endemicity of LD in the local area or in the area where the patient may have contracted the disease.
- Laboratory testing for lyme disease (LD) should be reserved for individuals with advanced manifestations that could represent late stage LD or in individuals from endemic areas with prolonged, unexplained flu-like symptoms (> 2wks) without erythema migrans because these individuals may have the early stage of the disease.
- Treatment of lyme disease should be tailored to the individual and the specific stage of the disease.

References

[1] Hayes E. Lyme disease. Clin Evidence 2001;497–504.
[2] CDC. Lyme disease - United States, 1999. MMWR 2001 50:181–5.
[3] Gerber MA, Zemel LS, Shapiro ED. Lyme arthritis in children: clinical epidemiology and long-term outcomes. Pediatrics 1998;102:905–8.
[4] Gerber MA. In: Rudolph AMM, Rudolph CD, editors. Rudolph's pediatrics. New York: McGraw-Hill Medical Publishing Division; 2002.
[5] Tugwell P, Dennis DT, Weinstein A, et al. Laboratory evaluation in the diagnosis of Lyme disease. Ann Intern Med 1997;127:1109–23.
[6] Berger BW, Johnson RC, Kodner C, et al. Cultivation of Borrelia burgdorferi from erythema migrans lesions and perilesional skin. J Clin Microbiol 1992;30:359–61.
[7] Smith R, Schoen R, Rahn D, et al. Clinical characteristics and treatment outcome of early Lyme disease in patients with microbiologically confirmed erythema migrans. Ann Intern Med 2002;136:421–8.
[8] Nadelman RB, Worsmer GP. Management of tick bites and early Lyme disease. In: Rahn DW, Evans J, editors. Lyme disease. Philadelphia: American College of Physicians; 1998. p. 49–76.
[9] Steere AC, Sikand VK. The presenting manifestations of Lyme disease and the outcomes of treatment. N Engl J Med 2003;348:2472–4.
[10] Rahn DW. Natural history of Lyme disease. In: Rahn DW, Evans J, editors. Lyme disease. Philadelphia: American College of Physicians; 1998. p. 35–48.
[11] Belman AL, Reynolds L, Preston T, et al. Cerebrospinal fluid findings in children with Lyme disease: associated facial nerve palsy. Arch Pediatr Adolesc Med 1997;151:1224–8.

[12] Eppes SC, Nelson DK, Lewis LL, et al. Characterization of Lyme meningitis and comparison with viral meningitis in children. Pediatrics 1999;103:957–60.

[13] Varde S, Beckley J, Schwartz I. Prevalence of tick-borne pathogens in Ixodes scapularis in a rural New Jersey county. Emerg Infect Dis 1998;4:97–9.

[14] Aguero-Rosenfeld ME. Laboratory aspects of tick-borne diseases: Lyme, human granulocytic ehrlichiosis and babesiosis. Mount Sinai J Med 2003;70:197–206.

[15] Sigal LH. Laboratory confirmation of the diagnosis of Lyme disease. Uptodate 2002;11.

[16] Bunikis J, Barbour AG. Laboratory testing for suspected Lyme disease. Med Clin North Am 2002;86:311–40.

[17] Jacobs RA. Infectious diseases: spirochetal. In: Tierney LM Jr, Papadakis MA, McPhee SJ, editors. Current medical diagnosis and treatment. 42nd edition. New York: McGraw-Hill; 2003.

[18] Ledue TB, Collins MF, Craig WY. New laboratory guidelines for serologic diagnosis of Lyme disease: evaluation of the two-test protocol. J Clin Microbiol 1996;34:2343–50.

[19] Johnson JB. Test approach and *Borrelia burgdorferi* strain selection for standardization of serodiagnosis of LD. In: Proceedings of the Second National Conference of Serologic Diagnosis of Lyme Disease. Washington, DC: Association of State and Territorial Public Health Laboratory Directors; 1994. p. 35–8.

[20] Qureshi MZ, New D, Zulqarni NJ, et al. Overdiagnosis and overtreatment of Lyme disease in children. Pediatr Infect Dis J 2002;21:12–4.

[21] Feder JHM, Hunt MS. Pitfalls in the diagnosis and treatment of Lyme disease in child. JAMA 1995;274:66–8.

[22] Bakken LL, Case K, Callister S, et al. Performance of 45 laboratories participating in a proficiency testing program for Lyme disease serology. JAMA 1992;268:891–5.

[23] Dattwyler RJ, Volkman DJ, Conaty SM, et al. Amoxycillin plus probenecid versus doxycycline for treatment of erythema migrans borreliosis. Lancet 1990;336:1404–6.

[24] Massorotti EM, Luger SW, Rahn DW, et al. Treatment of early Lyme disease. Am J Med 1992;92:396–403.

[25] Nadelman RB, Luger SW, Frank E, et al. Comparison of cefuroxime axetil and doxycycline in the treatment of early Lyme disease. Ann Intern Med 1992;117:273–80.

[26] Luger SW, Paparone P, Worsmer GP, et al. Comparison of cefuroxime axetil and doxycycline in treatment of patients with early Lyme disease associated with erythema migrans. Antimicrob Agents Chemother 1995;39:661–7.

[27] Luft BJ, Dattwyler RJ, Johnson RC, et al. Azithromycin compared with amoxicillin in the treatment of erythema migrans: a double-blind, randomized, controlled trial. Ann Intern Med 1996;124:785–91.

[28] Dattwyler RJ, Luft BJ, Kunkel MJ, et al. Ceftriaxone compared with doxycycline for the treatment of acute disseminated Lyme disease. N Engl J Med 1997;337:289–94.

[29] Worsmer GP, Ramanathan R, Nowakowski J, et al. Duration of antibiotic therapy for early Lyme disease: a randomized, double-blind, placebo-controlled trial. Ann Intern Med 2003;138:697–704.

[30] Klein MB, Nelson CM, Goodman JL. Antibiotic susceptibility of the newly cultivated agent of human granulocytic ehrlichiosis: promising activity of quinolones and rifamycins. Antimicrob Agents Chemother 1997;41:76–9.

[31] Dotevall L, Alestig K, Hanner P, et al. The use of doxycycline in nervous system Borrelia burgdorferi infection. Scand J Infect Dis 1998;53(Suppl):74–9.

[32] Dotevall L, Hagberg L. Successful oral doxycycline treatment of Lyme disease-associated facial palsy and meningitis. Clin Infect Dis 1999;28:569–74.

[33] Karlsson M, Hammers-Berggren S, Lindquist L, et al. Comparison of intravenous penicillin G and oral doxycycline for treatment of Lyme neuroborreliosis. Neurology 1994;44:1203–7.

[34] Hansen K, Hovmark A, Lebech AM, et al. Roxithromycin in Lyme borreliosis: discrepant results of an in vitro and in vivo animal susceptibility study and a clinical trial in patients with erythema migrans. Acta Derm Venereol 1992;72:297–300.

[35] Nowakowski J, McKenna D, Nadelman RB, et al. Failure of treatment with cephalexin for Lyme disease. Arch Fam Med 2000;9:563–7.

[36] Steere AC, Green J, Schoen RT, et al. Successful parenteral penicillin therapy of established Lyme arthritis. N Engl J Med 1985;312:869–74.

[37] Eichenfield AH, Goldsmith DP, Benach JL, et al. Childhood Lyme arthritis: experience in an endemic area. J Pediatr 1986;109:753–8.

[38] Steere AC, Levin RE, Molloy PJ, et al. Treatment of Lyme arthritis. Arthritis Rheum 1994;37:878–88.

[39] Schoen RT, Aversa JM, Rahn DW, et al. Treatment of refractory chronic Lyme arthritis with arthroscopic synovectomy. Arthritis Rheum 1991;34:1056–60.

[40] Logigian EL, Kaplan RF, Steere AC. Successful treatment of Lyme encephalopathy with intravenous ceftriaxone. J Infect Dis 1999;80:377–83.

[41] Bloom BJ, Wyckoff PM, Meissner HC, et al. Neurocognitive abnormlities in children after classic manifestations of Lyme disease. Pediatr Infect Dis J 1998;17:189–96.

[42] Klempner MS, Hu LT, Evans J, et al. Two controlled trials of antibiotic treatment in patients with persistent symptoms and a history of Lyme disease. N Engl J Med 2001;345: 85–92.

[43] Kaplan RF, Trevino RP, Johnson GM, et al. Cognitive function in post-treatment Lyme disease: do additional antibiotics help? Neurology 2003;60:1916–22.

Address reprint requests to

Andrew J. Foy, Jr., BS
Jefferson Medical College
950 Walnut Street, Apartment #416
Philadelphia, PA 19107-5596

e-mail: andrew.foy@jefferson.edu

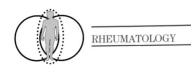
RHEUMATOLOGY   1522–5720/05 $15.00 + .00

LUPUS AND RELATED CONNECTIVE TISSUE DISEASES

Marcia L. Taylor, MD, and James M. Gill, MD, MPH

PRESENTATION AND PROGRESSION OF DISEASE

Cause and Pathology

Systemic lupus erythematosus (SLE) is an autoimmune disorder that affects multiple organ systems. The cause of the disease is unclear [1]. The hallmark of the disease is production of antibodies to the cell nucleus. These antibodies are referred to as antinuclear antibodies (ANA) and are seen in 95% of patients with SLE [2,3]. ANA are not unique to SLE and can occur in other autoimmune disorders, such as rheumatoid arthritis, scleroderma, mixed connective tissue disease, and polymyositis; ANA also occur in up to 5% of the normal population. Some patients with SLE may not have a positive ANA titer [3,4]. ANA bind to several different molecules in the nucleus, including DNA, RNA, histones, and small nuclear ribonucleoproteins. Antibodies to double-stranded DNA (anti-dsDNA) and to the Sm nuclear antigen (anti-Sm) are found only in patients with SLE [2,3].

The pathologic findings related to SLE are mainly related to inflammation and blood vessel abnormalities, including bland vasculopathy, vasculitis, and immune-complex deposition [2]. The pathologic findings of SLE-related nephritis are best understood and involve immune complex deposition in the glomerulus with anti-dsDNA playing a key role, which leads to the activation of the complement system [3]. Skin lesions demonstrate inflammation at the dermal-epidermal junction that is likely due to immune complex deposition and activation of the complement

From the Department of Family Medicine, Medical University of South Carolina, Charleston, South Carolina (MLT); and from the Department of Family and Community Medicine, Health Services Research, Christiana Care Health Services, Wilmington, Delaware (JMG)

pathway [2]. Autoantibodies may play a role in cytopenias that are often seen in SLE patients. Venous and arterial thrombosis is related to occlusive vasculopathy, which is related to general inflammation and inflammation in association with antiphospholipid and anticardiolipin antibodies and lupus anticoagulants [2,3].

SLE occurs in 1 in 2000 general outpatients and has an estimated general population prevalence of 40 to 50 per 100,000 [2,5]. The disease occurs more frequently in women between the ages of 15 and 40; there is a female-to-male ratio of 6 to 10:1 [2]. SLE shows a strong genetic component, with a 25% to 50% concordance rate in monozygotic twins and 5% in dizygotic twins and occurs with increased frequency in first-degree relatives [2,3]. Approximately 10% to 16% of patients with SLE have an affected first- or second-degree relative [6]. SLE more commonly affects African Americans than Caucasians, with prevalence rates in the United States being as high as 2.5 per 1000 in Native Americans, Hispanics, Asians, and African Americans [7].

Current research suggests that disturbances in the complement systems and B-cell function may predispose patients to the disease. Genome analysis has not shown an exact gene linkage, and current research suggests that multiple unlinked genes are involved in inducing SLE [3]. An association with human leukocyte antigen (HLA) has been found, with HLA-DR2 and HLA-DR3 being associated with a two- to five-time relative risk of SLE [2].

Environmental factors play a role in SLE. Ultraviolet B light has been implicated in flares of the disease [2,6,8]. It is estimated that approximately 70% of SLE patients have disease flare when exposed to UV light. Female sex hormones are felt to play a role in the disease, given the high female-to-male ratio and that pregnancy in many patients causes flares and worsens preexisting hypertension or nephritis [6,7]. Other studies have suggested an elevated risk for developing SLE in postmenopausal women treated with hormone replacement therapy and women using estrogen-containing oral contraceptives [9,10]. Infectious agents have been implicated as possible environmental factors that may lead to the development of SLE by inducing immune responses through molecular mimicry or by disrupting immunoregulation [2,6,7].

Several drugs are known to induce a SLE-like disease. Patients present frequently with arthritis, serositis, fatigue, fever, and positive ANA. Generally, these patients do not have nephritis or central nervous system (CNS) abnormalities and do not have positive anti-dsDNA or decreased complement levels. Symptoms usually disappear within a few weeks of stopping the drug and do not reoccur. Drugs that have been linked to drug-induced SLE include hydralazine, procainamide, isoniazid, hydantoin (eg, ethotoin and phenytoin), chlorpromazine, methyldopa, d-penicillamine, and minocycline. Patients who experience drug-induced SLE with one of these drugs should not be given the drug again. Rarely do these drugs cause flares in patients who have true SLE. Therefore, true SLE is not a contraindication for the use of these drugs [6].

Presentation

SLE affects multiple organ systems; therefore, patients may present with a variety of symptoms. The disease has a relapsing and remitting course and can be difficult to diagnosis in the early stages. Due to the wide variation in disease severity and organ systems affected, it is difficult to describe a typical presentation of SLE. Therefore, we discuss symptoms by organ system [7,11,12].

Constitutional symptoms such as fever, fatigue, weight loss, and general malaise are often early reported symptoms of SLE and occur in 70% to 85% of patients [7]. Arthritis and arthralgia, especially of the small joints of the hands and wrists, occur in 53% to 95% of patients [7]. The initial differential diagnosis for these symptoms is wide and includes systemic infection, malignancy, or other autoimmune disorders such as rheumatoid arthritis, Sjögren syndrome, and other connective tissue disorders.

Mucocutaneous symptoms are present in over 90% of SLE patients, and 4 of the 11 criteria for SLE are based on this fact [2]. The classic rash of SLE is the malar or butterfly rash, which occurs in 30% to 60% of patients [2]. This rash is erythematous and causes swelling over the bridge of the nose. It spreads to the malar eminences and classically spares the nasolabial folds. This rash is often exacerbated by exposure to sunlight and may leave postinflammatory pigmentary changes. Patients may exhibit erythematous rashes due to photosensitivity that do not meet criteria for the classic malar rash. SLE may present with other dermatologic manifestations, including discoid lupus and subacute cutaneous lupus erythematous, although these are seen less commonly [2,12]. Other mucocutaneous lesions of SLE include alopecia, which is generally diffuse and patchy. Alopecia is generally reversible, with hair regrowth beginning 6 to 8 weeks after flare resolution [1,2]. Ulcers are common and may occur in the mouth, nose, or anogenital area. Oral ulcers occur in 40% of patients [13] and are generally painless and occur on the hard palate, tongue, buccal mucosa, and gingival surfaces [1].

Arthralgias and arthritis are common in patients with SLE. Unlike rheumatoid arthritis, SLE arthritis is generally nonerosive and non-deforming, although it involves similar areas, including the metacarpophalangeal joints, wrists, and metatarsophalangeal joints. Some patients with SLE have deformities of their joints (referred to as Jaccoud arthropathy), but these are generally reducible and are due to involvement of the para-articular tissues [2,6].

The kidney is commonly affected in SLE. Renal involvement (lupus nephritis) is present in 50% of all patients and in 75% of African American patients [12]. Lupus nephritis has a wide range of severity, and the World Health Organization (WHO) has classified lupus nephritis based on histologic examination of the kidney after renal biopsy. The WHO categories are normal, mesangial, focal and segmental proliferative, diffuse proliferative, and membranous lupus nephritis. Diffuse proliferative and progressive forms of focal proliferative nephritis are associated with worse outcomes than membranous or mesangial nephritis [2]. Nephrotic syndrome (proteinuria of over 3.5 g/d, hypoalbuminemia, hyperlipidemia, and edema) or renal failure may be the presenting signs of lupus nephritis. Many authorities recommend that patients with SLE have annual serum creatine and urinalysis to monitor for proteinuria, hematuria, pyuria, and casts in the absence of infection to monitor renal function [2,12]. Finally, certain categories of lupus nephritis are associated with certain auto-antibodies. For example, proliferative glomerulonephritis is associated with ds-DNA antibodies, and membranous glomerulopathy is associated with Smith antibodies. Renal involvement may be seen in association with any auto-antibodies. [6]

Neuropsychiatric symptoms occur in 66% of patients with SLE and can involve the peripheral, central, and autonomic nervous systems. Clinical symptoms include headache, seizures, stroke, cranial (usually optic) and peripheral neuropathies, psychosis, depression, transverse myelitis, Guillain-Barré syndrome, and cognitive function abnormalities [2,6,12]. It is important to exclude other causes (eg, infection) as the cause of the patient's symptoms. MRIs of patients with SLE have shown small, diffuse involvement of the white or gray matter, which is believed to indicate that microemboli are associated with the neuropsychiatric symptoms [6,12].

SLE affects the cardiovascular system. Pericarditis is common, occurring in approximately 25% of patients [2]. Most effusions are small to moderate and respond to treatment with corticosteroids. Valvular disease is another cardiac manifestation of SLE, with many patients requiring valve replacement surgery. The aortic valve is most commonly affected, possibly due to fibrosis, valvulitis, bacterial endocarditis, aortitis, or Libman-Sacks endocarditis. Libman-Sacks involves verrucous vegetations on the cardiac valves that are not due to infectious causes. Prophylactic subacute bacterial endocarditis treatment is recommended for all patients with SLE before dental or surgical procedures (grade of recommendation: D) [2]. Another important cardiovascular complication is premature or accelerated atherosclerosis, which represents a major cause of morbidity and mortality. This is believed to be due to an affect of SLE and its treatment. Six percent to 10% [14] of patients with SLE have premature atherosclerosis; this number approaches 40% in screening studies [15,16]. Therefore, screening for other cardiovascular risk factors (eg, smoking, hyperlipidemia, and hypertension) is important in patients with SLE. Another cardiovascular complication with SLE is thrombosis. This is due to the formation of antiphospholipid antibodies such as anticardiolipin and lupus anticoagulant. Thrombosis increases the likelihood of venous and arterial thrombosis and spontaneous abortion. Approximately 30% to 50% of patients with SLE form antiphospholipid antibodies [12].

Hematologic abnormalities are present in SLE. Anemia is often present and may be due to chronic disease, medication side effects, or peripheral destruction. Anemia is present in about 80% of patients, with less than 10% having a true autoimmune hemolytic anemia [2]. Leukopenia occurs in 50% of patients and is usually a lymphopenia rather than a neutropenia [2]. Thrombocytopenia and an elevated erythrocyte sedimentation rate may be present. In patients with active disease flares, complement levels such as C3 and C4 may be depressed. Positive ANA titers occur in over 99% of SLE patients at some point in the disease [17,18]. A titer of 1:40 or higher is the most sensitive diagnostic criteria [5].

Other rheumatologic diseases and healthy patients may have a positive ANA. Therefore, a positive ANA titer should not be considered diagnostic of SLE. Following ANA titers in patients with known SLE is not useful because ANA titers do not track the severity of flares. Anti-dsDNA occurs in approximately 40% of SLE patients; anti-dsDNA has a 95% specificity for SLE and correlates with disease activity and renal involvement [2,13]. Anti-Sm occurs in 30% of patients and is highly specific for SLE [13]. Anti-Ro (SS-A) and -La (SS-B) antibodies are seen in SLE and are associated with dry mouth, photosensitivity, neonatal lupus, and congenital heart block. Anti-RNP may be seen in SLE and is associated with musculoskeletal symptoms, although it may be seen in patients with mixed connective tissue disorder. Finally, antihistone antibodies may be seen in SLE patients, although they are more likely to be associated with drug-induced lupus [2,13]. Table 1 lists the clinical features of SLE.

Diagnosis

The diagnosis of SLE is based on history and physical and laboratory findings. The American College of Rheumatology (ACR) has established criteria for the diagnosis of SLE. Recent studies have found these criteria to be 78% to 96% sensitive and 89% to 96% specific for SLE [17,18,36,37]. To diagnose SLE, 4 of the 11 criteria must be met serially or simultaneously during any period of observation (grade of recommendation: B). Box 1 lists the diagnostic criteria for SLE [18–20].

Elevation of the ANA titer levels of 1:40 or greater is seen in 99% of patients with SLE and is the most sensitive diagnostic criteria [5,17,18]. Positive ANA levels may be seen in 5% of healthy patients and in other hematologic diseases, including Sjögren syndrome (68% of patients have a positive ANA), scleroderma (40% to 75%), and rheumatoid arthritis (25% to 50%) [35]. Titers in these patients are generally lower than those of patients with SLE. Due to the high false-positive rate of ANA in primary care patients where the prevalence of SLE is lower, the ACR recommends performing ANA testing only in patients who have two or more unexplained signs and symptoms that are listed in Table 1 (grade of recommendation: D) [5,17,21]. A consistently negative ANA can be assumed to exclude the diagnosis of SLE. A patient with a negative ANA with organ system involvement of SLE should be evaluated for an alternative diagnosis; if no other cause is found, the patient should be referred to a rheumatologist for evaluation for ANA-negative SLE. If a patient with a previous negative ANA develops new clinical symptoms consistent with SLE, the ACR recommends repeat ANA testing (grade of recommendation: D). Laboratory testing for anti-dsDNA and anti-Sm may

TABLE 1.
Clinical Features of Systemic Lupus Erythematosus

System	Signs/Symptoms
Constitutional	Fatigue, fever (in the absence of infection), weight loss
Musculoskeletal	Arthritis, arthralgia, myositis
Skin	Butterfly rash, photosensitive rash, mucous membrane lesion, alopecia, Raynaud phenomenon, purpura, urticaria, vasculitis
Renal	Hematuria, proteinuria, casts, nephrotic syndrome
Gastrointestinal	Nausea, vomiting, abdominal pain
Pulmonary	Pleurisy, pulmonary hypertension, pulmonary parenchymal disease
Cardiac	Pericarditis, endocarditis, myocarditis
Reticuloendothelial	Lymphadenopathy, splenomegaly, hepatomegaly
Hematologic	Anemia, thrombocytopenia, leukopenia
Neuropsychiatric	Psychosis, seizures, organic brain syndrome, transverse myelitis, cranial neuropathies, peripheral neuropathies

Adapted from American College of Rheumatology Ad Hoc Committee on Systemic Lupus Erythematosus Guidelines. Guidelines for referral and management of systemic lupus erythematosus in adults. Athritis Rheum 1999;42:1785–96; with permission.

be useful in patients who have a positive ANA but do not meet full SLE diagnostic criteria. These tests are highly specific for SLE but are not very sensitive. Therefore, a positive result for one of these tests helps to establish the diagnosis of SLE, but a negative result does not rule out SLE [5,17,21]. ACR guidelines recommend rheumatologic referral for patients with symptoms of SLE and positive ANA, especially if these patients have more than mild or stable disease (grade of recommendation: D) [21]. Fig. 1 shows an algorithm for the diagnosis of SLE.

NATURAL HISTORY AND TREATMENT

The management of SLE is challenging because the management of disease symptoms must be balanced against the adverse side effects of the medications used in treatment. In general, therapy is individualized, and the intensity is determined by the severity of SLE, with mild disease requiring symptomatic treatment and more severe life-threatening or organ-threatening disease requiring more aggressive treatment. Patient education about SLE and its unpredictable course plays an important part in treatment [21]. Many patient educational resources are available from the ACR, the Arthritis Foundation, and the Lupus Foundation of America

---

Box 1. 1997 Revised/Revised Classification Criteria for Systemic Lupus Erythematosus

Before a patient can be classified as having definite SLE, at least four of the following 11 disorders must be present at some time in the disease course:

- Malar rash: fixed erythema, flat or raised, over the malar eminences, tending to spare the nasolabial folds
- Discoid rash: erythematous raised patches with adherent keratotic scaling and follicular plugging
- Photosensitivity: unusual skin rash due to reaction to sunlight, by patient history or physician observation
- Oral ulcers: oral or nasopharyngeal ulceration, usually painless, observed by physician
- Arthritis: nonerosive arthritis involving two or more peripheral joints, characterized by swelling, tenderness, or effusion
- Serositis: pleuritis by convincing history or pleuritic pain or rub heard by a physician or evidence of pleural effusion OR pericarditis documented by EKG, rub, or evidence of pericardial effusion
- Renal disorder: persistent proteinuria ›0.5 g per day or ›3+ or cellular casts, which may be red cell, hemoglobin, granular, tubular, or mixed
- Neurologic disorder: seizures or psychosis in the absence of offending drugs or known metabolic derangements (uremia, ketoacidosis, or electrolyte imbalance)
- Hematologic disorder: hemolytic anemia with reticulocytosis, OR leukopenia ‹4000/mm^3 on two or more occasions, OR lymphopenia ‹1500/mm^3 on two or more occasions, OR thrombocytopenia ‹100,000/mm^3 in the absence of offending drugs
- Immunologic disorder: positive anti-phospholipid antibody or anti-dsDNA antibody or anti-Sm antibody or false-positive serologic syphilis test known to be positive for at least 6 months and confirmed by negative Treponema pallidum immobilization or fluorescent treponemal antibody absorption test
- Antinuclear antibodies: an elevated titer of antinuclear antibody by immunofluorescence or an equivalent assay at any point in time and in the absence of drugs known to be associated with "drug-induced lupus" syndrome

Adapted from Tan EM, Cohen AD, Fries JF, et al. The 1982 revised criteria for the classification of systemic lupus erythematosus. Arthritis Rheum 1982;25:1274, with permission; and Hochberg MD. Updating the American College of Rheumatology revised criteria for the classification of systemic lupus erythematosus. Arthritis Rheum 1997;40:1725, with permission.

---

[1]. Several lifestyle modifications must be discussed. Due to the photosensitive rash with SLE, the ACR recommends that patients avoid prolonged sun exposure and use sunscreen regularly (grade of recommendation: D). Two randomized clinical control trials have shown the benefits of topical glucocorticoid creams in treating the cutaneous

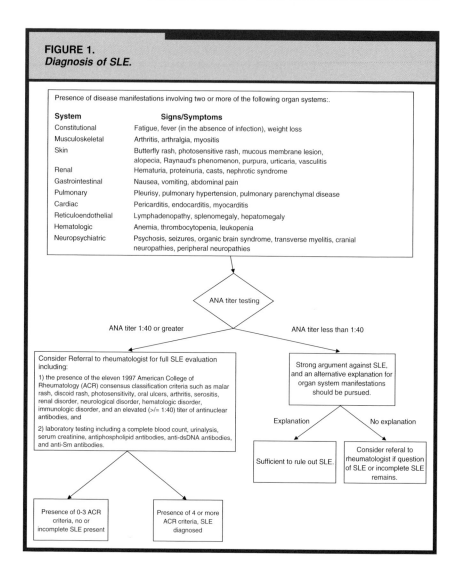

FIGURE 1.
Diagnosis of SLE.

Presence of disease manifestations involving two or more of the following organ systems:.

System	Signs/Symptoms
Constitutional	Fatigue, fever (in the absence of infection), weight loss
Musculoskeletal	Arthritis, arthralgia, myositis
Skin	Butterfly rash, photosensitive rash, mucous membrane lesion, alopecia, Raynaud's phenomenon, purpura, urticaria, vasculitis
Renal	Hematuria, proteinuria, casts, nephrotic syndrome
Gastrointestinal	Nausea, vomiting, abdominal pain
Pulmonary	Pleurisy, pulmonary hypertension, pulmonary parenchymal disease
Cardiac	Pericarditis, endocarditis, myocarditis
Reticuloendothelial	Lymphadenopathy, splenomegaly, hepatomegaly
Hematologic	Anemia, thrombocytopenia, leukopenia
Neuropsychiatric	Psychosis, seizures, organic brain syndrome, transverse myelitis, cranial neuropathies, peripheral neuropathies

ANA titer testing

ANA titer 1:40 or greater — ANA titer less than 1:40

Consider Referral to rheumatologist for full SLE evaluation including:

1) the presence of the eleven 1997 American College of Rheumatology (ACR) consensus classification criteria such as malar rash, discoid rash, photosensitivity, oral ulcers, arthritis, serositis, renal disorder, neurological disorder, hematologic disorder, immunologic disorder, and an elevated (>/= 1:40) titer of antinuclear antibodies, and

2) laboratory testing including a complete blood count, urinalysis, serum creatinine, antiphospholipid antibodies, anti-dsDNA antibodies, and anti-Sm antibodies.

Strong argument against SLE, and an alternative explanation for organ system manifestations should be pursued.

Explanation — No explanation

Sufficient to rule out SLE.

Consider referal to rheumatologist if question of SLE or incomplete SLE remains.

Presence of 0-3 ACR criteria, no or incomplete SLE present

Presence of 4 or more ACR criteria, SLE diagnosed

manifestations of SLE (grade of recommendation: A) [22,23]. High-dose glucocorticoid creams should be avoided on areas of the skin that are prone to atrophy, such as the face. The ACR recommends that patients be educated to seek early medical attention with any unexplained fevers (grade of recommendation: D). Infections are common in SLE and are the leading cause of death, accounting for approximately 33% of all deaths [11]. The ACR recommends aggressive monitoring and treatment for modifiable cardiovascular risk factors, such as hypertension, hyperlipidemia, tobacco use, sedentary lifestyle, and obesity, due to the increased risk of cardiovascular disease seen in SLE (grade of recommendation: D).

Patients should have routine health maintenance, gynecologic examinations, and immunizations for hepatitis B, *Haemophilus influenzae*, Pneumovax, and influenza per ACR recommendations (grade of recommendation: D) [21].

Nonsteroidal anti-inflammatory agents (NSAIDs) have been examined in the treatment of SLE for musculoskeletal symptoms, especially those related to joint pain, pleuritis, pericarditis, and headache. Two recently published reviews of the current evidence on the effectiveness of NSAIDs use in SLE determined that NSAIDs were effective, but these studies were mainly case reports and retrospective studies with small sample sizes (grade of recommendation: C) [24,25]. The adverse side effects of NSAIDs include gastrointestinal (GI) bleeding, renal toxicity, hepatic toxicity, and worsening of hypertension and peripheral edema. In one trial investigating NSAIDs use in SLE, aseptic meningitis was noted in some patients given ibuprofen [26]. The ACR recommends baseline complete blood count (CBC), creatinine, urinalysis, liver enzymes, yearly CBC, and creatinine with chronic NSAIDs therapy (grade of recommendation: D). The use of selective cyclooxygenase (COX)-2 inhibitors has not been studied in SLE, although it is theorized that the GI side effects with these agents may be less than with traditional NSAIDs [2]. Careful consideration should be used with COX-2 agents due to the recent increased risk of cardiovascular disease seen with rofecoxib [27].

Corticosteroids are another mainstay of SLE treatment. Topical corticosteroids are often used to treat the cutaneous manifestations of SLE. Fluocinonide cream has been shown to be more effective than hydrocortisone cream for discoid lupus in two randomized clinical trials (grade of recommendation: A) [22,23]. Intra-articular corticosteroids have been suggested as treatment for arthritis symptoms; however, most of the studies examining their utility have not examined patients with SLE (grade of recommendation: D) [2]. Systemic corticosteroids are used at varying dosages and routes of administration depending on the severity of symptoms. Symptoms that are treated with corticosteroids include constitutional symptoms, arthritis, serositis, nephritis, cerebritis, vasculitis, and hematologic abnormalities. Low doses of corticosteroids (generally less than 10 mg/d) [1] may be use to treat constitutional symptoms of mild arthritis and arthralgias. If the patient requires increased dosages of the steroids, the patient may need more aggressive therapy, such as with antimalarial agents. Most of the research with corticosteroids in SLE has been as open-labeled trials and case reports (grade of recommendation: C).

Corticosteroids have been studied in high dosages for severe SLE symptoms. Randomized clinical control trials and a meta-analysis of randomized clinical control trials have demonstrated corticosteroids to be beneficial in the treatment of severe CNS disease, glomerulonephritis, thrombocytopenia, and hemolytic anemia [22,28–31]. Life-threatening organ involvement, including nephritis, cerebritis, systemic vasculitis, and hematologic abnormalities, require high doses of oral corticosteroids (1–2 mg/kg/d) or parental steroids. In very severe cases, up to 1 g of methylprednisolone may be administered for 3 consecutive days [21]. Current guidelines suggest that for severe CNS disease, nephritis, thrombocytopenia, and hemolytic anemia, large doses of corticosteroids and other immunosuppressive agents should be used as therapy (grade of recommendation: A) [22]. There are many side effects of corticosteroid treatment, including weight gain, emotional liability, osteonecrosis, hypertension, hyperlipidemia, diabetes, glaucoma, osteoporosis, and increased risk of infections. Current ACR guidelines recommend baseline blood pressure, bone density, glucose, potassium, lipid profile, yearly lipid and bone density studies, and checking the urine every 3 to 6 months for any patient who is on chronic corticosteroids (grade of recommendation: D) [21]. Patients should never have their corticosteroid therapy stopped abruptly; rather, it should be tapered down gradually because adrenal suppression may occur with chronic use. Patients treated with more than 20 mg/d of prednisone for at least 1 month will have some degree of adrenal suppression. Adrenal suppression can occur with as little as 20 to 30 mg/d of prednisone for 5 days, but adrenal function rapidly returns to normal after prednisone is discontinued. When tapering the dose of prednisone, doses greater than 40 mg/d can be tapered at a dose of 10 mg/wk, and doses between 20 and 40 mg/d can be tapered at 5 mg/wk. For doses less than 20 mg/d, tapering may be best managed by patient-dictated schedules by dosing alternate days before reducing the total daily dosage (grade of recommendation: D) [2].

Antimalarials represent another class of medications that have been examined in the treatment of SLE. Antimalarials include hydroxychloroquine, chloroquine, and quinacrine. These agents treat the constitutional, cutaneous, and musculoskeletal symptoms, although their effects in preventing long-term organ damage are not clearly understood [2,22]. These agents help to decrease the dosage of steroids needed for adequate control of symptoms and may be used in combination when one agent is not effective in controlling symptoms. One 24-week randomized clinical control trial of hydroxychloroquine showed that there was a 2.5 times greater increased risk of disease flares in patients who discontinued the drug than in those who continued on it (grade of recommendation: A) [31]. Hydroxychloroquine is believed to have the additional benefits of lowering low-density lipoproteins and anti-thrombotic effects. Antimalarials are generally well tolerated by patients, and their side effects are generally mild and include headache, myalgia, rash, and GI upset. Their most concerning side effect is that of ophthalmologic toxicity, although this is rare with the relatively low doses that are used in SLE treatment [2]. Current ACR guidelines recommend baseline ophthalmologic examination and then every 6 to 12 months while on the medication (grade of recommendation: D) [21].

Several immunomodulating agents have been examined in SLE, including azathioprine, cyclophosphamide, methotrexate, chlorambucil, cyclosporine, and nitrogen mustard, with selection of the agent depending on the patient's symptoms [21]. These agents should be prescribed in consultation with a rheumatologist. Azathioprine works by inhibiting nucleic acid synthesis as a purine analog and affects humoral and cellular immunity. Azathioprine is used mainly to treat nephritis and as a steroid sparing agent in the treatment of other SLE symptoms [2]. In the treatment of nephritis, some studies have shown that azathioprine with cortico-steroids may not be as effective as cyclophosphamide with corticosteroids [32–35]. Either treatment is superior to corticosteroids alone for nephritis. A recent Cochrane meta-analysis of randomized clinical control trials of azathioprine with corticosteroids for the use in SLE nephritis showed a decrease in overall mortality but not in renal outcomes (grade of recommendation: A) [36]. Azathioprine may cause bone marrow and GI toxicity and an increase in malignancy rate, including non-Hodgkin lymphoma. Dosage adjustment is needed with renal or hepatic impairment [2]. Baseline CBC, creatinine, and liver enzymes are recommended along with CBC every 1 to 2 weeks with any dosage change and then every 1 to 3 months thereafter. Yearly liver enzymes and pap tests are recommended by the ACR (grade of recommendation: D) [21].

Cyclophosphamide has been examined in the treatment of SLE with severe organ involvement, especially nephritis. The use of this drug in the treatment of nephritis has been well studied [37]. The best response rates in treatment have occurred in patients with diffuse proliferative lupus nephritis. Cyclophosphamide may also be used in the treatment of cytopenia, CNS disease, pulmonary hemorrhage, and vasculitis. A recent Cochrane meta-analysis of randomized clinical control trials of cyclo-phosphamide and corticosteroids showed a decrease in renal complica-tions but not in overall mortality (grade of recommendation: A) [36]. Cyclophosphamide has serious side effects, including gonadal toxicity, myelosuppression, myeloproliferative disorders, hemorrhagic cystitis, and malignancy, including bladder cancer [21]. Current ACR recommen-dations are for baseline CBC with differential and urinalysis and monthly CBC and urinalysis and yearly urine cytology and pap smears (grade of recommendation: D) [21]. Any patient on this drug who presents with hematuria should be referred to a urologist for cystoscopic evaluation.

Methotrexate has been recently examined in the treatment of mild SLE, although it has not been studied as extensively as other agents. One double-blind, randomized, clinical trial has examined the use of metho-trexate in SLE and has found that doses of 15 to 20 mg/wk for a total of 6 months controlled disease symptoms, especially cutaneous and muscu-loskeletal symptoms, and helped to reduce the dose of corticosteroids needed (grade of recommendation: A) [38]. Side effects of therapy include myelosuppression, hepatic fibrosis, and pulmonary fibrosis. Current guidelines recommend a baseline CBC, chest x-ray, creatinine, liver function tests, and hepatitis panels followed by CBC, liver enzymes, creatinine, and urinalysis every 4 to 8 weeks (grade of recommendation: D) [21].

Cyclosporine has been used in the treatment of SLE and has its mechanism of action by inhibiting the T-cell–mediated response [2]. Cyclosporine has been used to address the renal manifestations of SLE, especially membranous nephritis or refractory nephrotic syndrome [2]. Although few controlled studies exist on this subject, one recent literature review of cyclosporine therapy showed that it decreased overall disease activity (grade of recommendation: C) [39]. Side effects of the drug include hypertension, mild elevation in creatinine, and gingival hyperplasia. Mycophenolate mofetil, which inhibits purine synthesis, has shown promise in the treatment of lupus nephritis, especially diffuse proliferative glomerulonephritis [2].

Several other types of therapy have been investigated in SLE with varying results. Bromocriptine has been examined in the treatment of SLE even in the absence of hyperprolactinemia, with one randomized clinical trial showing good results (grade of recommendation: A) [40]. Dehydroepiandrosterone has been examined in the treatment of mild to moderate SLE and with other drugs for the treatment of more severe symptoms including nephritis, serositis, and hematologic problems; one recent review of the literature of controlled and uncontrolled trials showed the drug to have benefit in SLE (grade of recommendation: B) [41]. Danazol has been examined in the treatment of hematologic abnormalities, with one observational uncontrolled study showing benefit (grade of recommendation: C) [42]. Thalidomide has been examined for the treatment of discoid lupus, with one observational study showing benefit [43], although the side effects of peripheral neuropathy and severe birth defects limit its use (grade of recommendation: C) [2]. Dapsone has been examined in the treatment of discoid lupus, with observational case reports showing benefit (grade of recommendation: C) [30] Topical retinoids have been used in the treatment of cutaneous lupus, with a randomized clinical control trial showing benefit (grade of recommendation: A) [44]. Patients who have a thrombotic event require long-term anticoagulation therapy with warfarin with a target International Normalized Ratio of 3 to 4 as determine by a large retrospective cohort study (grade of recommendation: B) [16]. Table 2 provides a summary of the medications, their recommended uses, and level of evidence.

Plasmapheresis has been examined in the treatment of SLE, although it has serious side effects, such as increased risk of infection, anaphylaxis, and high cost of the procedure. Plasmapheresis is thought to work by removing circulating immune complexes and antibodies. This therapy is believed to play a role in cryoglobulinemia, hyperviscosity syndrome, and thrombotic thrombocytopenia purpura. The role of plasmapheresis in the treatment of lupus nephritis remains controversial. Intravenous immunoglobulin has also been studied in the treatment of SLE and has been noted to improve symptoms of thrombocytopenia, arthritis, nephritis, fever, mucocutaneous symptoms, and immunologic function. Side effects of therapy include fever, headache, myalgia, arthralgia, and rarely aseptic meningitis [2]. A thorough discussion of these two treatments is beyond the scope of this article.

Even with optimal treatment, some patients with SLE nephritis progress to end-stage renal disease and require dialysis and possibly renal transplant. The recurrence rate of SLE nephritis in transplanted kidneys is

TABLE 2.
Medications, Recommended Uses, and Level of Evidence

Medication	Targeted Symptoms	Grade of Recommendation
Topical glucocorticoids	Cutaneous	A
Systemic glucocorticoids	Constitutional, musculoskeletal, serositis, nephritis, vasculitis, cerebritis, hematologic	A for life-threatening complications, C for milder symptoms
Anti-malarials	Constitutional, cutaneous, musculoskeletal	A
Azathioprine	Nephritis, steroid-sparing agent	A
Cyclophosphamide	Nephritis, vasculitis, pulmonary, CNS. Generally for life-threatening organ involvement	A
Methotrexate	Cutaneous musculoskeletal	A
Cyclosporine	Nephritis	C
Bromocriptine	Decrease disease flares in combination with other medications	A
Dehydroepiandrosterone	Nephritis, serositis, hematologic	B
Danazol	Hematologic	C
Thalidomide	Discoid lupus	C
Dapsone	Discoid lupus	C
Topical retinoids	Discoid lupus	A

6% [45]. One study reported that rejection rates were higher than those of the general population of kidney transplant recipients [45], whereas another study showed little difference in rejection rates [46].

There are some new experimental therapies that are being evaluated for the treatment of SLE. Some of these therapies involve immunosuppressive agents that are more specific in their action than current therapies. These new agents are able to target specific pathways needed for T-cell/B-cell activation, the production of anti-dsDNA antibodies, and cytokine activation. The possibility of autologous hematopoietic stem-cell transplantation is also being evaluated [2].

In conclusion, SLE is a disease with a variable course and manifestations that can affect a variety of organ systems. Family medicine physicians have an important role in the recognition of the early signs and symptoms of SLE and in the initial diagnosis. Although mild SLE may be managed by the primary care physician, many patients require referral to a rheumatologist for more aggressive management of their symptoms, especially with life-threatening organ involvement.

Key Points

- SLE is a multisystem autoimmune disorder of unknown etiology that affects mainly women of childbearing age.
- SLE is characterized by the production of auto-antibodies such as ANA, anti-dsDNA, anti-Sm, and antiphospholipid antibodies.
- The diagnosis of SLE is made if patients have four or more of the 11 criteria for SLE according to the ACR criteria.
- Patients with SLE are at an increased risk for cardiovascular disease.
- A variety of pharmacologic agents are used in the treatment of SLE. The choice of which agent is dependent upon the patient's symptoms, with milder disease responding to low-dose corticosteroids and nonsteroidal anti-inflammatory agents. More severe disease requires the use of immunomodulating therapies with rheumatology referral.

References

[1] Dall'Era M, Davis JC. Systemic lupus erythematosus. Postgrad Med 2003;114:31–7, 40.
[2] Klippel JH, Crofford LJ, Stone JH, et al, editors. Primer on the rheumatic diseases. 12th edition. Atlanta: Arthritis Foundation; 2001. p. 329–52, 593–8.
[3] Criscione LG, Pisetsky DS. The pathogenesis of systemic lupus erythematosus. Bull Rheum Dis 2004;52. Available at: http://www.arthritis.org/research/bulletin/vol52no6/printable.htm. Accessed October 26, 2004.
[4] Gomella LG, editor. Clinician's pocket reference. 8th edition. Stamford: Appleton & Lange; 1997. p. 48–9.
[5] Gill JM, Quisel AM, Rocca PV, et al. Diagnosis of systemic lupus erythematosus. Am Fam Physician 2003;68:2179–86.
[6] Ruddy S, Harris ED, Sledge CB, editors. Kelley's textbook of rheumatology. 6th edition. Philadelphia: W.B. Saunders; 2001. p. 1089–152.
[7] Systemic lupus erythematosus—first consult Available at: www.firstconsult.com/home/us_disorder/01014951/part1.htm. Accessed October 29, 2004.
[8] Wysenbeek AJ, Block DA, Fries JF. Prevalence and expression of photosensitivity in SLE. Rheumatol Dis 1989;48:461–3.
[9] Sanchez-Guerrero J, Liang MH, Karlson EW, et al. Postmenopausal estrogen therapy and the risk of developing systemic lupus erythematosus. Ann Intern Med 1995;122:430–3.
[10] Sanchez-Guerrero J, Karlson EW, Liang MH, et al. Past use of oral contraceptives and the risk of developing systemic lupus erythematosus. Arthritis Rheum 1997;40:804–8.
[11] Ferri FF, editor. Practical guide to the care of the medical patient. 6th edition. St. Louis: Mosby; 2004. p. 810–3.
[12] Rakel RE. Textbook of family practice. 6th edition. Philadelphia: W.B. Saunders; 2002. p. 978–82.
[13] Koopman WJ, editor. Arthritis and allied conditions. 14th edition. Baltimore: Lippincott Williams & Williams; 2001. p. 1455–71.
[14] Petri M, Perez-Gutthann S, Spence D, et al. Risk factors for coronary artery disease in patients with systemic lupus erythematosus. Am J Med 1992;93:513–9.
[15] Petri M. Treatment of systemic lupus erythematosus: an update. Am Fam Physician 1998;57:2753–60.
[16] Khamashta MA, Cuadrado MJ, Mujic F, et al. The management of thrombosis in the antiphospholipid-antibody syndrome. N Engl J Med 1995;332:993–7.

[17] Gilboe IM, Husby G. Application of the 1982 revised criteria for the classification of systemic lupus erythematosus on a cohort of 346 Norwegian patients with connective tissue disease. Scand J Rheumatol 1999;28:81–7.

[18] Tan EM, Cohen AS, Fries JF, et al. The 1982 revised criteria for the classification of systemic lupus erythematosus. Arthritis Rheum 1982;25:1271–7.

[19] Gladman D, Ginzler E, Goldsmith C, et al. The development and initial validation of the systemic lupus international collaborating clinics/American College of Rheumatology damage index for systemic lupus erythematosus. Arthritis Rheum 1996;39:363–9.

[20] Hochberg MC. Updating the American College of Rheumatology revised criteria for the classification of systemic lupus erythematosus [letter]. Arthritis Rheum 1997;40:1725.

[21] American College of Rheumatology Ad Hoc Committee on Systemic lupus Erythematosus Guidelines. Guidelines for referral and management of systemic lupus erythematosus in adults. Arthritis Rheum 1999;42:1785–96.

[22] National Guideline Clearinghouse. Available at: www.guideline.gov. Accessed October 19, 2004.

[23] Jessop S, Whitelaw D, Jordaan F. Drugs for discoid lupus erythematosus. Cochrane Database Syst Rev 2001;1:CD002954.

[24] Ostense M, Villiger PM. Nonsteroidal anti-inflammatory drugs in systemic lupus erythematosus. Lupus 2000;9:566–72.

[25] Ostense M, Villiger PM. Nonsteroidal anti-inflammatory drugs in systemic lupus erythematosus. Lupus 2001;10:135–9.

[26] Hawkey CJ, Karrasch JA, Szczepanski L, et al. Omeprazole compared with misoprostol for ulcer associated with nonsteroidal antiinflammatory drugs: Omeprazole versus Misoprostol for NSAID-Induced Ulcer Management (OMNIUM) Study Group. N Engl J Med 1998;338:727–34.

[27] Study connects Vioxx to heart attack and stroke, Merck issues voluntary withdrawal. Available at: www.home.mdconsult.com/das/news. Accessed November 23, 2004.

[28] Boumpas DT, Austin HA, Vaughn EM, et al. Controlled trial of pulse methylprednisolone versus 2 regimens of pulse cyclophosphamide in severe lupus nephritis. Lancet 1992;340: 741–5.

[29] Bansal VK, Beto JA. Treatment of lupus nephritis: a meta-analysis of clinical trials. Am J Kidney Dis 1997;29:193–9.

[30] Avina-Zubieta JA, Galindo-Rodriguez G, Robledo I, et al. Long-term effectiveness of danazol corticosteroids and cytotoxic drugs in the treatment of hematologic manifestations of systemic lupus erythematosus. Lupus 2003;12:52–7.

[31] The Canadian Hydroxychloroquine Study Group. A randomized study of the effect of withdrawing hydroxychloroquine sulfate in systemic lupus erythematosus. N Engl J Med 1991;324:150–4.

[32] Boumpas DT, Fessler BJ, Austin HA III, et al. Systemic lupus erythematosus: emerging concepts: part 2. Dermatologic and joint disease, the antiphospholipid antibody syndrome, pregnancy and hormonal therapy, morbidity, and mortality, and pathogenesis. Ann Intern Med 1995;123:42–53.

[33] Boumpas DT, Fessler BJ, Austin HA III, et al. Systemic lupus erythematosus: emerging concepts. Part 1. Renal, neuropsychiatric, cardiovascular, pulmonary and hematologic disease. Ann Intern Med 1995;122:940–50.

[34] Hahn BH, Kantor OS, Osterland CK. Azathioprine plus prednisone versus prednisone alone in the treatment of systemic erythematosus: a report of a prospective, controlled trial in 24 patients. Ann Intern Med 1975;83:597–605.

[35] Steinberg AD, Steinberg SC. Long term preservation of renal function in patients with lupus nephritis receiving treatment that includes cyclophosphamide versus those treated with prednisone only. Arthritis Rheum 1991;34:945–50.

[36] Flanc RS, Roberts MA, Strippoli GF, et al. Treatment for lupus nephritis. Cochrane Database Syst Rev 2004;1:CD002922.

[37] Ortmann RA, Klippel JH. Update on cyclophosphamide for systemic lupus erythematosus. Rhematol Dis Clin North Am 2000;26:363–75.

[38] Carneiro JR, Sato EI. Double blind, randomized, placebo controlled clinical trial of methotrexate in systemic lupus erythematosus. J Rheumatol 1999;26:1275–9.

[39] Hallegua D, Wallace DJ, Metzger AL, et al. Cyclosporine for lupus membranous nephritis: experience with ten patients and review of the literature. Lupus 2000;9:241–51.

[40] Alvarez-Nemegyei J, Cobarrubias-Cobos A, Escalante-Triay F, et al. Bromocriptine in systemic lupus erythematosus: a double-blind, randomized, placebo-controlled study. Lupus 1998;7:414–9.

[41] van Vollenhoven RF. Dehydroepiandrosterone in systemic lupus erythematosus. Rheum Dis Clin North Am 2000;26:349–62.

[42] Cervera H, Jara LJ, Pizarro S, et al. Danazol for systemic lupus erythematosus with refractory autoimmune thrombocytopenia or Evans' syndrome. J Rheumatol 1995;22: 1867–71.

[43] Atra E, Sato EI. Treatment of the cutaneous lesions of systemic lupus erythematosus with thalidomide. Clin Exp Rheumatol 1993;11:487–93.

[44] Ruzicka T, Sommerburg C, Goerz G, et al. Treatment of cutaneous lupus erythematosus with acitretin and hydroxychloroquine. Br J Dermatol 1992;127:513–8.

[45] Stone JH, Milward CL, Olson JL, et al. Frequency of recurrent lupus nephritis among ninety-seven renal transplant patients during the cyclosporine era. Arthritis Rheum 1998;41:678–86.

[46] Ward MM. Outcomes of renal transplantation among patients with end-stage renal disease caused by lupus nephritis. Kidney Int 2000;57:2136–43.

Address reprint requests to

Marcia L. Taylor, MD
Department of Family Medicine
Medical University of South Carolina
PO Box 250192, 295 Calhoun Street
Charleston, SC 29425

e-mail: taylo@musc.edu

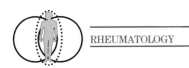
POLYMYALGIA RHEUMATICA AND GIANT CELL ARTERITIS

John A. Donnelly, MD, and Seth Torregiani, DO

Polymyalgia rheumatica (PMR) is a systemic inflammatory disease that occurs in patients older than 50 years of age and is characterized by an elevated erythrocyte sedimentation rate (ESR), proximal extremity pain, morning stiffness, and rapid relief with the administration of cortico-steroids. Giant cell arteritis (GCA), also known as temporal arteritis or Horton disease, is an inflammatory vasculitis of large and medium vessels primarily arising from the aortic arch. It occurs in adults older than 50 years of age and is characterized by headache, jaw claudication, and visual loss.

PMR and GCA are frequently discussed together due to their well-known association [1,2]. Many experts consider the two diseases to be two points along a continuum of a specific systemic inflammatory disease syndrome, with PMR being the expression of a milder form of disease and GCA suggesting more severe disease [1]. As evidence, experts point to findings of similar HLA expression [2] in the two conditions and the presence of increased levels of specific cytokines common to both. Although these findings are somewhat controversial, there is an undeniable link between the two diseases (Table 1).

Both conditions are diseases of the elderly population, occurring exclusively in persons over 50 years of age and peaking in incidence between 70 and 80 years of age [1]. Both conditions occur most frequently in Caucasians, particularly those of northern European descent and those living at higher latitudes [1,3–5]. Further strengthening the link between PMR and GCA are population-based studies demonstrating a 16% to 21% incidence of GCA in patients with PMR, whereas symptoms consistent with PMR can been seen in 40% to 60% of persons with GCA [1].

Patients with PMR should be evaluated for clinical signs of GCA, and vice versa. Despite these connections, the workup and treatment of each

From the Department of Internal Medicine and Pediatrics, Christiana Care Health Systems, Newark, Delaware

TABLE 1.
Comparison of Polymyalgia Rheumatica and Giant Cell Arteritis

Polymyalgia Rheumatica	Giant Cell Arteritis
Age >50	Age >50
Women 2:1	Women 2:1
Incidence 58/100,000	Incidence 25/100,000
Most common in persons of northern European descent	Most common in persons of northern European descent
16% to 21% have comorbid GCA	40% to 60% have comorbid PMR
Interleukin-6 elevated	Interleukin-6 elevated
Responds quickly to corticosteroids	Responds quickly to corticosteroids

Abbreviations: GCA, giant cell arteritis; PMR, polymyalgia rheumatica.

condition may vary for physicians considering these diagnoses. Much of the research and many of the publications address individual aspects of each condition. For these reasons, this article addresses each disease entity separately.

POLYMYALGIA RHEUMATICA

Epidemiology

Isolated PMR occurs at an incidence of 58.7 per 100,000 persons aged 50 years or older, according to a 30-year population-based study performed in Olmstead County, Minnesota [6]. The majority of cases of PMR occur in women: 67% of cases in the Olmstead County study were women, consistent with the 2:1 female-to-male incidence of PMR found in other population-based studies [6–8]. The mean age at presentation of PMR was 72.8 years [6,7], and incidence increases with advancing age beyond 50 years. Incidence peaks between 70 and 79 years of age in women and beyond 80 years of age in men, after which the incidence begins to decline [6,7]. PMR occurs more often in Caucasians than in any other racial or ethnic group. Caucasians of Northern European descent are most often affected, suggesting a possible genetic predisposition to the disease.

PMR does not confer increased mortality. Multiple studies have demonstrated that mortality rates among both sexes affected by PMR are no greater than those of the general population [6–8].

Pathophysiology

Various mechanisms have been postulated as causes of PMR, but the exact etiology is unclear. PMR most likely results from a genetic vulnerability combined with environmental factors to trigger a systemic inflammatory response in the patient [1].

Symptoms of PMR often develop rapidly, and some studies have demonstrated a seasonal variation in its incidence [9], leading some experts to postulate an infectious trigger for PMR. Multiple infectious etiologies have been implicated, including parainfluenza virus type 1 [10,11], mycoplasma pneumoniae [12], parvovirus B19 [13], and others [1]. Other studies have called into question the seasonal distribution of PMR or a correlation with infectious vectors [14–16].

The precise factors that give rise to the characteristic pain and stiffness of the proximal muscles in PMR are uncertain. There are frequently no consistent pathologic findings in muscle, and vasculitis may or may not be present in isolated PMR [3]. Nonspecific markers of inflammation, including ESR and C-reactive protein (CRP), are elevated, suggesting that a systemic inflammatory syndrome is responsible for the clinical manifestations of PMR. There is also evidence to suggest that the inflammatory manifestations of PMR are cytokine mediated (as opposed to T-cell mediated) [17]. Interleukin (IL)-6 levels are elevated in patients with PMR, and plasma concentrations of IL-6 correlate with clinical symptoms and disease severity. Furthermore, IL-6 levels decrease rapidly in response to corticosteroid administration. Steroids do not seem to suppress the underlying mechanism leading to increased production of IL-6 [17].

The large, proximal joints of the body (hip and glenohumeral) frequently exhibit a non-erosive synovitis [18], and a tenosynovitis can be seen in the biceps tendon, wrist flexor, or extensor tendons [19]. Knee and ankle effusions are also seen [19]. Inflammation of proximal bursae, including the subacromial and subdeltoid bursae [20,21] and the iliopectineal bursae of the hip [22], is also often present and may further explain the classic proximal pain distribution, which is one of the hallmarks of PMR [21]. One of the distinguishing characteristics of PMR is the presence of extracapsular inflammation, a finding that may help distinguish it from rheumatoid arthritis or other arthritides [23].

Clinical Presentation

PMR most often presents clinically with aching pain and stiffness of the proximal extremities in a person over 50 years of age (Box 1). In an Olmstead County, Minnesota study [7], the shoulders were the most commonly affected area. Shoulder pain and stiffness occurred in 94% of study participants with PMR, followed by the hips (nearly 80%), neck (63%), and torso (40%). Symptoms are characteristically worse in the morning [7,18]. The onset of PMR is acute, and the musculoskeletal symptoms most often present bilaterally, although they may initially present unilaterally and become bilateral as the disease progresses [3]. Often, the symptoms have been present for >1 month before coming to a physician's attention.

Box 1. Clinical Features of PMR

- Bilateral synovitis of large proximal joints; shoulders > hips
- Peripheral joint involvement possible but less severe
- Subacromial and iliopectineal bursitis common
- Morning stiffness > 1 hour
- Acute onset, often progressing over 1 month before diagnosis
- Constitutional symptoms common
- Full range of motion and normal strength testing

In addition to the classic proximal limb complaints, PMR can present with distal extremity manifestations. One study found that 20% of patients with PMR presented with a nondeforming mono- or oligoarticular arthritis of the distal joints, including the knees, wrists, metacarpophalangeal joints, interphalangeal joints, sternoclavicular joints, and elbow [18]. One case series noted that distal extremity swelling with pitting edema (occurring in 8% of patients), which was believed to result from a tenosynovitis of the distal extremities, may be an overlooked manifestation of PMR [25]. In isolated PMR, distal symptoms are not seen in the absence of proximal symptoms [18]. Thirty percent of patients may also complain of constitutional, "flu-like" symptoms including malaise, fatigue, anorexia, weight loss, and low-grade fever. Some patients may also report depression [7].

On physical examination, patients may demonstrate tenderness over affected areas and limited active range of motion. Full passive range of motion and normal strength is typically present [26,27].

Laboratory Findings

The classic laboratory finding in PMR is an ESR >40 mm/h. Elevation of the ESR is the only published laboratory criterion for diagnosing PMR [1,28,29] and has a sensitivity of 80% for the disease [30]. Despite this, two retrospective studies have found that as many as 20% of patients with PMR may present with a normal or only mildly elevated ESR ($\leq$40 mm/h) [31,32].

A normal ESR in the setting of a clinical diagnosis of PMR may indicate a milder form of disease [32], although the clinical presentation and duration of symptoms and treatment is similar to patients with PMR and elevated ESR. Such patients may take longer to come to clinical attention due to the persistently "normal" ESR. In such cases, a CRP level may be useful. CRP, an acute phase reactant, is also typically elevated in PMR (normal value <0.5 mg/dL) [1], and one study has demonstrated that CRP is more sensitive than ESR in assessing disease activity at diagnosis of PMR. An elevated CRP is not considered part of the published diagnostic criteria for PMR.

Although they are not commonly used in the office setting, levels of IL-6 are elevated in PMR and may be useful in further distinguishing patients with symptoms of PMR and a normal ESR. A mild normocytic, normochromic anemia may be present. Liver enzymes may be elevated in approximately 25% of patients, particularly alkaline phosphatase [28]. CK levels are normal [26].

Diagnosis

The diagnosis of PMR is made primarily by using clues from a thorough history and physical examination. A number of experts have empirically developed clinical criteria to aid in the diagnosis [1].

Chuang et al [28] and Healey [29] have proposed similar diagnostic criteria for PMR. These include age >50 years; bilateral aching stiffness of the shoulders, neck, or pelvic girdle for >1 month; morning stiffness lasting longer than 1 hour; an ESR >40 mm/h; and the absence of any other disease, except GCA, that may cause similar symptoms, such as polymyositis or rheumatoid arthritis. Healey [29] adds an additional criterion: prompt response to daily treatment with at least 20 mg of prednisone. Failure to achieve a prompt and complete response to corticosteroid therapy should initiate a search by the clinician for a different cause of the symptoms, such as another rheumatic condition or an occult malignancy.

According to a *New England Journal of Medicine* review [1] of PMR and GCA, all of the previously mentioned criteria must be present to make the diagnosis of PMR. Since these criteria were developed, retrospective data have been published revealing that up to 20% of patients with a clinical diagnosis of PMR may have a normal ESR. Chuang et al's [28] criteria were developed based on findings from a 10-year period (1970–1979) during the Olmstead County, Minnesota epidemiologic study of PMR, whereas Healey's [29] criteria were developed from a case series (grade of recommendation for the use of these clinical criteria: B) [29]. Diagnostic imaging methods such as MRI or ultrasonography are not usually obtained in the evaluation of PMR but may aid in the diagnosis of patients with a normal ESR by demonstrating typical findings, such as non-erosive or nondestructive synovitis of the glenohumeral or hip joints (versus the typical erosive synovitis seen in rheumatoid arthritis) [33].

The differential diagnosis of PMR is broad (Box 2). The disorder can generally be distinguished from other diseases on the basis of clinical presentation, laboratory evaluation, response to steroid therapy, or diagnostic imaging. Diseases that can mimic PMR include polymyositis, drug-induced myopathies (eg, statins), hypothyroid myopathy, systemic lupus erythematosus, rheumatoid arthritis or other arthritides, bacterial endocarditis, fibromyalgia, depression, cervical or lumbar radiculopathies, bilateral rotator cuff injury, and various malignancies or paraneoplastic syndromes [26,34].

Treatment

Corticosteroids are the cornerstone of treatment of PMR. The usual starting dose of prednisone is 10 to 20 mg/d [3].This is continued for

---

Box 2. Differential Diagnosis of PMR

- Myopathy: drug induced, hypothyroid, polymyositis
- Systemic lupus erythematosus
- Rheumatoid arthritis
- Fibromyalgia
- Bilateral cervical radiculopathy
- Bilateral rotator cuff injury
- Paraneoplastic syndromes
- Depression

---

1 month and is carefully tapered by 1 to 2.5 mg/mo to a dosage of 10 mg/d, based on clinical response [3,27]. The dosage may be further tapered by 1 mg every 4 to 6 weeks to a maintenance dose of 5 to 7.5 mg/d [27].

There are no randomized, controlled trials demonstrating the efficacy of corticosteroids. Numerous epidemiologic, prospective, and retrospective studies have consistently shown corticosteroids to be the treatment of choice in PMR [1,6–8,18,35] (grade of recommendation: B).

Discontinuation of steroids may be attempted after 6 to 12 months if the ESR has normalized and the patient is symptom free. This is usually accomplished by continuing to taper the dosage by 1 mg every 6 to 8 weeks. Most patients require treatment for 3 to 6 years. Relapses are most common in the first 18 months of therapy [27].

Patients should be monitored for complications of long-term steroid therapy, including osteoporosis, adrenal insufficiency, diabetes/hyperglycemia, hypertension, cataracts, glaucoma, and increased susceptibility to infection [3]. Because patients are exposed to corticosteroids for months to years, all patients should be considered for calcium replacement and bisphosphonates at the time corticosteroids are initiated. Diabetics need close monitoring and medication adjustments as corticosteroid doses are changed.

Weyand et al [35] have attempted to identify patients who may require lower dosages of steroids and a shorter course of treatment based on initial laboratory findings and clinical presentation. In their prospective study, patients fell into one of three subgroups. Group A included patients with an initial lower ESR (<50 mm/h) and IL-6 level (<10 pg/mL) and rapid response to prednisone at 10 mg daily, group B included patients with a higher ESR (>50 mm/h) and IL-6 level (>10 pg/mL) who had a good initial response to prednisone therapy at 20 mg/d but had frequent relapses and required chronic therapy, and group C included patients with elevated lab values but higher levels of disease activity and a poor initial response to 20 mg/d of prednisone. Patients in group C required an increase in their dosage of prednisone to 30 mg/d or a longer treatment period at 20 mg and a higher chronic dosage of prednisone in the first 6 months of treatment [35].

Although the number of participants in this study was small ($n = 27$), the results suggest that with further study there may be criteria to identify patients with PMR who will do well on lower doses or shorter courses of therapy but will still have a durable response to prednisone, sparing them potential long-term complications of steroid treatment (group A). Such criteria may identify patients (those in groups B or C) who require more aggressive initial therapy or a longer course of treatment to control their disease.

Based on the findings from this study, the authors made initial recommendations for the management of PMR based on the three strata of disease severity. These guidelines require further clarification before they can be put into daily clinical practice. Based on the authors' conclusions, patients in group A can be treated with 10 mg of prednisone daily, and the dose can be reduced by 1 mg every month, with a short course of disease expected. Patients in group B require an initial dose of prednisone of 20 mg/d, which can be reduced by 2.5 mg weekly after improvement of symptoms to 10 mg/d, followed by 1 mg reductions each month. An intermediate course of disease (>12 months) can be expected, with exacerbation of symptoms if the dose of prednisone is lowered too quickly. Patients in group C require an initial prednisone dose of 20 mg for 2 to 4 weeks, with dose adjustment based on symptom control and normalization of IL-6 levels. In this subgroup of patients, a prolonged disease course with relapse can be expected (grade of recommendation: B).

Methotrexate has been studied as a potential steroid-sparing agent for the long-term treatment of PMR. The results have been inconclusive, and only two randomized controlled trials have addressed this question. The first found no benefit to the addition of methotrexate to prednisone in PMR [36]. A more recent randomized trial showed a potential benefit, but the improvement with methotrexate was small [37], and an accompanying editorial questioned whether the benefit outweighed the difficulties inherent in methotrexate therapy [38]. Therefore the addition of methotrexate to prednisone is not standard of care for PMR, and further study is needed to determine whether this is a viable approach (grade of recommendation: D).

GIANT CELL ARTERITIS

Epidemiology

GCA is an inflammatory vasculitis of large and medium vessels primarily arising from the aortic arch. Although it can be seen in variety of populations, there is an epidemiologic predilection for people of northern European decent and those living at higher latitudes [4]. Women are twice as likely to be affected as men. Cases are rare before 50 years of age, and incidence increases with age, peaking in the eighth decade [1]. The United States incidence is 15 to 25 per 100,000 in adults over 50 years of age [2] and peaks at 1100 per 100,000 persons 85 year of age [39].

Pathophysiology

Although the etiology of GCA is unknown, epidemiologic studies suggest a potential relationship between multiple environmental and genetic factors. There is a specific ethnic group and region of the globe with the highest incidence of GCA. Studies have suggested a seasonal variation and cyclical variations with peak incidence every 5 to 7 years [40]. These studies have prompted investigation into an infectious cause. Studies have looked at links between mycoplasma pneumoniae, para-influenza virus, parvovirus B19, varicella zoster virus, and chlamydia pneumoniae [13,41–43]. Although many of these small studies have been suggestive of infectious etiology, no definitive research has shown a causative organism.

Cytokine production is clearly associated with the vascular inflammation. Cytokine production is likely related to a cell-mediated process. The result is vascular infiltrate with lymphocytes, macrophages, and multinucleated giant cells [44].

Inflammation may be patchy within the vessels arising from the aortic arch, most commonly the branches of the external carotid artery, such as the temporal artery [1]. The inflammatory lesions result in intimal thickening and arterial narrowing. Thrombosis at sites of narrowing is possible, and effected patients often develop areas of ischemia or infarction. The inflammatory vascular lesions that cause the greatest morbidity are located within the vessels supplying the optic nerve and retina [45]. The visual consequences of vasculitis within this blood supply are discussed elsewhere.

Clinical Presentation

GCA has a variable clinical expression, so practitioners must be familiar with the range of symptoms to help raise awareness of the diagnosis (Table 2). Clinical signs can help direct diagnostic testing.

Systemic symptoms—particularly, fatigue, malaise, anorexia, and fever—are common. Prolonged fever without a source in older adults should raise suspicion for temporal arteritis and prompt investigation into other clinical and laboratory manifestations [46]. "Silent" GCA has been characterized as patients with GCA but with no localized symptoms. In a series of 175 biopsy-proven patients with GCA, 21 patients had no localized symptoms, and 14 patients met criteria for a fever of unknown origin. There was an association between presentation with "silent" GCA and an extremely elevated ESR and CRP and lower hemoglobin. No patients without localized symptoms of cranial vasculitis progressed to permanent visual loss [47]. A Spanish study found 10% of patients with GCA presented with fever. A more intense inflammatory response with higher ESR and lower hemoglobin had a negative association with ischemic events [48]. Thus, silent GCA arteritis is less likely to progress to visual loss or cranial ischemia.

TABLE 2.
Clinical Features of Giant Cell Arteritis

Symptom	Percentage of Patients
New onset headache	65
Jaw claudication	39
Diplopia	11
Amaurosis fugax	11
Scalp tenderness	41
Fever	42
Weight loss	43
Vertigo	11

Data from Hunder GG, Bloch DA, Michel BA, et al. The American College of Rheumatology 1990 criteria for the classification of giant cell arteritis. Arthritis Rheum 1990;33:1122–9.

Systemic symptoms may be in the form of PMR. Any patients with classic PMR symptoms should be evaluated for clinical signs of GCA, such as localized headache, jaw claudication, and visual disturbances. Routine biopsy of PMR patients without clinical manifestations of GCA is not recommended [49].

Headache is the most common clinical manifestation, with two thirds of patients experiencing this symptom during the course of illness [50]. Headache can occur in any region of the head but tends to be localized in the region of the temporal artery. The occipital artery may be involved, creating posterior headache. A more specific marker for GCA is the complaint of scalp pain rather than actual headache; this is found in 40% of patients [51]. New-onset headache or scalp pain in any patient over 50 must years of age raise clinical suspicion of GCA.

Jaw claudication, found in 40% of patients, is one of the most specific signs of GCA [51]. This symptom is generally characterized as fatigue and pain of the muscles of mastication. The pain is most notable when the patient eats food that requires prolonged mastication, such as tough meat or bread. Patients may experience a similar symptom from prolonged talking or singing. Claudication may present as tongue pain or chronic odynophagia. Necrotic lesions of the tongue progressing to complete necrosis within a few days have been reported in the literature [52].

Some patients may present with a reduction in jaw opening width [53]. This is thought to occur from the same mechanism as jaw claudication, with partial ischemia in the muscles of mastication. Other rare oral manifestations can include maxillary pain, dysphagia, dry cough, and hoarseness [54]. Facial artery involvement may present as facial pain. A rare case of submandibular mass has been reported [55].

Undiagnosed visual symptoms can create the most long-term morbidity for patients with GCA. Initial presentation may be of transient visual loss or amaurosis fugax. Early suspicion and treatment of GCA in patients with transient visual symptoms can prevent progression to complete vision loss.

Diplopia may be an early manifestation of GCA that occurs from vasculitic lesions causing ischemia of the lateral eye muscles [56]. Patients may note persistent diplopia or may note it only on lateral gaze. Diplopia, found in just over 10% of patients, is one of the more specific findings for GCA and should raise suspicion in any patient with this symptom over 50 years of age. GCA should be considered in patients over 50 years of age who present with cranial nerve neuropathies with the appearance of a third, fourth, or sixth nerve palsy [56].

Permanent visual loss occurs in approximately 15% of patients with GCA [57]. Blurring, diplopia, or amaurosis fugax occurs in 65% of patients before the development of permanent visual loss [58]. The progression to permanent visual loss has been found to occur in an average of 8.5 days after these early findings. Therefore, early work-up and treatment can help protect against permanent problems [50]. Initially, permanent visual loss may present as a partial visual field cut. This visual loss may progress to complete unilateral or bilateral vision loss within days of presentation. Physical examination of the effected eye may show a pale and swollen disc or retinal hemorrhage. This occurs when the retinal arteries, the ophthalmic artery, or the posterior ciliary arteries are affected with vasculitic lesions [45].

Although the most common presentation of GCA involves the extracranial arteries of the head and neck, vasculitis may develop in other vessels of the aortic arch. One study of 168 patients found that 27% of patients with GCA arteritis had large artery involvement [59]. This group of patients was found to have stenosis of the cervical or subclavian arteries resulting in arm claudication symptoms. Large-vessel involvement has been found to be more common in women and in a slightly younger age group, with a mean age of presentation of 66 [60]. A negative association with classic cranial symptoms and the development of large vessel complications were found [53].

Aortic arch involvement can result in serious consequences. In a study with a group of 96 patients with GCA, it was found that 10% developed thoracic aortic aneurysm. It took a median of 5.8 years after diagnosis of GCA for the aneurysms to be detected. Abdominal aortic aneurysm was found in 5% of patients an average of 2.5 years after diagnosis. When compared with age-matched control subjects, patients with GCA are 17.3 times more likely to develop a thoracic aortic aneurysm and 2.4 times more likely to develop an abdominal aortic aneurysm [61]. In two separate studies, fatal thoracic aorta dissection occurred in 50% of patients with aneurysm [53,55].

Despite the lack of intracranial vasculitis, cerebrovascular accidents are a documented complication of GCA. They likely occur from vasculitis, thrombosis, and emboli formation from lesions in the internal carotids and vertebral arteries. An association between CVA and the presence of jaw claudication and visual loss has been noted [62]. Although vasculitis of the coronaries was not documented, a retrospective Swedish study found a higher incidence rate of cardiovascular events in patients with GCA [63]. Other rare findings in GCA have included biopsy-proven vasculitis in the breast, iliacs, and diaphragmatic paralysis from cervical radicular vessels [59,64,65]. Other recent studies have shown an association between GCA and the classic symptoms of benign positional vertigo [66].

Laboratory Findings

GCA has some classic laboratory findings that should be known by practitioners. Most of these are typical of inflammatory conditions.

ESR is a well-known marker for inflammatory conditions, including GCA. Most patients with GCA have an ESR >50 mm/h. Although GCA studies have not established a well-defined "normal" ESR, past studies have suggested a value of age/2 for men and [age + 10]/2 for women [67,68]. With this in mind, a normal ESR is uncommon in GCA. A 2002 meta-analysis found that only 4% of patients with biopsy-proven GCA had "normal" ESR [68]. A study of patients diagnosed between 1950 and 1998 found only 9 of 167 patients had an ESR of <40 [69]. As a nonspecific marker of inflammation, ESR >50 has a reported specificity of 48% [51].

CRP is another commonly used inflammatory marker. A small study found that CRP was >6 mg/L in 49 of 55 cases of GCA [70]. There is conflicting literature on the accuracy of CRP or ESR to diagnose and follow GCA, with some authors favoring CRP and some favoring ESR [63,71,72]. Using both studies together may be helpful; one series found that 1% of patients with biopsy-proven GCA had a normal CRP and a normal ESR [40].

More recent research has looked at the use of thrombocytosis in the evaluation of temporal arteritis. One series found a mean platelet count of 433,000 for patients with biopsy positive arteritis and a mean count of 277,000 for patients with a negative biopsy [73]. Another small study of patients presenting with optic neuropathy found a correlation between patients presenting with thrombocytosis and the eventual biopsy-proven GCA [74]. Most recently, a study did not find thrombocytosis to be more accurate at predicting GCA than ESR, but it did find a higher predictive value when both were elevated [65].

The presence of normocytic, normochromic anemia is another helpful tool. Although pooled data have shown only 44% sensitivity for positive biopsy [61], anemia can be helpful when evaluating disease activity. Studies have shown a negative correlation between the presence of anemia and the likelihood to progress to ischemic complications, such as permanent vision loss [40].

Other commonly abnormal labs include microscopic hematuria in one third of patients [75], increased hepatic transaminase and alkaline phosphatase in one third of patients [45], and anticardiolipin antibodies in 50% of patients [76]. Although they are not often available for clinical use, elevated levels of interleukin-6 seem to have a positive correlation with disease activity [17].

The differential diagnosis of GCA depends on the presenting symptom (Box 3). New-onset headache should raise suspicion for intracranial mass or subdural hematoma. Diplopia should raise suspicion for cranial nerve neuropathies. Jaw claudication should raise suspicion of temporomandibular joint arthritis. Visual loss may be caused by optic neuropathy or cerebrovascular disease. Rarely, polyarteritis nodosa causes cranial symptoms [77]. Takayasu arteritis can cause aortic or upper extremity symptoms.

Diagnosis

Biopsy of the temporal artery is the gold standard for the diagnosis of GCA. However, only 10% to 30% of temporal arteries biopsied are proven to be consistent with temporal arteritis. Therefore, using the clinical clues to help direct biopsy in a patient with cranial or visual symptoms is essential.

In a 2002 meta-analysis, only 39% of biopsies for suspected GCA confirmed the diagnosis [61]. This meta-analysis determined which clinical sign can help direct toward a positive biopsy. The researchers found that jaw claudication is found in only 34% of patients with GCA but is the most specific historical clue. Another study found that the combination of jaw claudication with diplopia was 100% specific for positive biopsy [78]. No historical clues have been found to carry a high negative predictive value (grade of recommendation: A).

Objective data can help to guide biopsy. On physical examination, abnormalities of the temporal artery, such as enlargement, pain, beading, or loss of pulse, carried the highest likelihood ratios of 4.3, 4.6, 2.7, and 2.6, respectively (Table 3) [68]. The presence of synovitis makes the likelihood of GCA low and should prompt investigation into an alternate diagnosis. The use of an elevated ESR was not found to be a specific finding with a likelihood ratio of 1.1. An elevated ESR has been found to be sensitive: ESR values listed as abnormal, >50, or >100 were listed with sensitivities of 96%, 83%, and 39%, respectively (Table 4).

Box 3. Differential Diagnosis of GCA

- Cranial vasculitis: Takayasu arteritis, polyarteritis nodosa
- New onset headache in patient > 50 years of age: intracranial mass, subdural hematoma
- Diplopia: cranial neuropathy, diabetes mellitus
- Jaw claudication: temporomandibular joint arthritis
- Vision loss: optic neuropathy, cerebrovascular accident

TABLE 3.
Likelihood Ratio of Giant Cell Arteritis Using Physical Examination Findings

Examination Finding	Likelihood Ratio
Beaded temporal artery	4.6
Enlarged artery	4.3
Tender artery	2.6
Pulseless artery	2.7
Scalp tenderness	1.6
Synovitis	0.4

Data from Smentana GW, Shmerling RH. Does this patient have temporal arteritis? JAMA 2002;287;92–101.

In summary, elevated ESR is one of the most sensitive markers, and jaw claudication, diplopia, and abnormal temporal artery are the most specific. One study found age that the combination of age >70 years, new headache, jaw claudication, and abnormal temporal artery examination has a positive predictive value of 100% [79]. Another study found that patients who had synovitis without claudication, temporal artery abnormalities, and ESR >31 had a 95% probability of having a negative temporal artery biopsy [80]. The use of ESR to assist in the diagnosis of GCA is recommended (grade of recommendation: A).

The use of duplex ultrasound to assist in the diagnosis of GCA has been considered by a number of small studies. Findings on ultrasound include dark halo around the lumen of the temporal artery and segmental stenosis or occlusions of temporal arteries [81]. A diagnostic study of 89 patients in 2002 found that the presence of a hypoechoic halo had a sensitivity of only 40% and a specificity of 79% [82]. This found that the use of ultrasound was not more useful than using clinical clues to direct

TABLE 4.
Sensitivity of Erythrocyte Sedimentation Rate in Giant Cell Arteritis

ESR	Sensitivity
>age/2	96%
>50	83%
>100	39%

Abbreviation: ESR, erythrocyte sedimentation rate.
Data from Evans JM, O'Fallon WM, Hunder GG. Increased incidence of aortic aneurysm and dissection in giant cell (temporal) arteritis: a population-based study. Ann Intern Med 1995;122:505–7.

biopsy. Alternatively, another small study found that by using halo or stenosis on ultrasound, the sensitivity, specificity, positive predictive value, and negative predictive value were 100%, 80%, 58%, and 100%, respectively [83]. Two studies have found that the use of ultrasound of the occipital arteries in patients with symptoms of occipital artery involvement has a sensitivity of 65% and a specificity approaching 100% [84,85]. Until more consistent evidence shows that ultrasound is more helpful then clinical clues in the diagnosis of GCA, the current recommendation is to not make a biopsy decision based on ultrasound findings.

Other imaging modalities have been investigated, including CT, MRI, PET, and gallium scanning. Early case reports looked promising for PET scanning; however, a more recent study of 22 patients did not show utility [86,87]. Two small preliminary studies have found correlation with the increased uptake in the temporal artery distribution and a positive biopsy when using gallium scanning [88,89].

Biopsy remains the standard for diagnosis of GCA and should be performed in any patient with a high suspicion of GCA. Positive biopsy findings typically show granulomatous inflammation of the vessel wall with infiltration of multinucleated giant cells, macrophages, and T cells. Biopsy may only carry a 90% to 95% sensitivity at predicting which patients go on to require corticosteroid treatment [90,91]. Therefore, some patients with convincing clinical presentation should be treated with corticosteroids regardless of biopsy result.

The length of biopsy specimen has been debated in the literature. The segmental inflammation has led some authors to suggest sampling 3 to 5 cm of temporal artery, whereas others believe 1 to 2 cm is adequate. Pathologic examination of multiple levels of the biopsied artery helps increase the sensitivity of the procedure [92]. It seems that biopsy of a clinically abnormal temporal artery requires a smaller sample size.

There has been debate on unilateral versus bilateral biopsy for the most accurate diagnosis. Two recent studies found that only 1% of patients with a negative unilateral biopsy had a positive contralateral biopsy [93,94]. Other studies have found that 2.4% to 3% of patients had a negative biopsy followed by a positive contralateral biopsy [70]. Because of this controversy, many surgeons follow the 1983 recommendation of taking a 3.5-cm biopsy from one side and contralateral biopsy only if the first is negative on frozen section [45,83]. Until evidence conclusively finds that unilateral biopsy is as good as bilateral in finding GCA, the current recommendation is to use caution and continue to follow the 1983 recommendations (grade of recommendation: D).

The rapid progression of visual loss has prompted many physicians to start treatment before temporal artery biopsy is obtained. A number of studies have shown that accuracy of biopsy is not affected within a few weeks of initiating corticosteroid treatment [95,96]. Therefore, if there is a high clinical suspicion of GCA, there is a continued recommendation to treat with corticosteroids even if a biopsy has not been obtained (grade of recommendation: B).

Treatment

The mainstay of treatment in GCA has been glucocorticoids. Timing and dosing of corticosteroids has been debated for a number of years. In response to the morbidity caused by long-term systemic steroid exposure, more recent research has looked into corticosteroids sparing medication regimens. Because the use of glucocorticoids in the treatment of GCA has been so well established, there will likely never be a placebo-controlled trial of glucocorticoids (grade of recommendation: B).

Prompt treatment of GCA is essential for the preservation of visual function. Once visual symptoms occur, rapid progression to irreversible and sometimes complete visual loss is common. Therefore, studies have looked at the appropriate initial dose of steroids to preserve visual function. No large controlled trials comparing high-dose pulse intravenous steroids to low or moderate oral steroids have been performed. Two recent studies have shown conflicting results regarding initial high-dose intravenous steroids to preserve visual function.

A 2001 retrospective study of 73 biopsy proven cases of GCA patients with visual loss found using variable high-dose intravenous regimens that there was a 40% likelihood of improved vision, compared with a 13% likelihood in patients treated with oral steroids [97]. The initial steroid regimens in this study varied from 1000 mg/d of methylprednisolone for 3 days to 250 mg methylprednisolone twice daily for 3 or more days. Average initial oral steroid dose was not well characterized in the study.

A 2003 retrospective study of 32 patients with visual loss and biopsy-proven GCA found improved visual acuity in only five patients after treatment with high-dose intravenous steroids [98]. The steroid regimen used was 250 mg of intravenous methylprednisolone every 6 hours for 3 days followed by 1 mg/kg of oral prednisone for 4 weeks. All five of the patients who had some visual improvement were found to have clinically significant restriction of the visual fields resulting in significant long-term morbidity.

A randomized controlled trial of 164 patients looked at the overall long-term outcome after initial therapy with high-dose intravenous methylprednisolone [99]. Patients were randomized to receive 0.7 mg/kg/d of oral prednisone or a 240 mg intravenous dose of methylprednisolone followed by 0.5 to 0.7 mg/kg/d oral prednisone. The researchers did not find significant differences in long-term treatment outcomes or overall steroid dose after 1 year.

Other studies have looked at outcomes when a patients weres started on low-dose oral steroids. A number of retrospective studies have found that an initial steroid dose of 10 to 20 mg/d of oral prednisone has equal long-term outcomes when compared with higher doses of medication [100–102]. There were no significant differences in the development of visual complication between the groups. A more recent retrospective study found that starting patients at lower initial doses resulted in lower maintenance doses, with year 2 doses averaging 4.1 mg/d [103]. One study found that patients started on <40 mg/d had a higher relapse of clinical symptoms, and the required doses needed to be increased to keep symptoms controlled [104]. Until evidence on the starting dose of glucocorticoids is better established, the recommendation is to continue with the established practice of initiating at 40 to 60 mg/d (grade of recommendation: D).

Because the average GCA patient requires 24 or more months of corticosteroid treatment, side effects are common. A number of studies have looked at treatment regimens that can reduce the total corticosteroid burden. Most of this research has involved the use of methotrexate as an adjuvant treatment.

Two randomized, placebo-controlled studies enrolling 21 and 98 patients looked at the benefit of adding methotrexate to patients on corticosteroids [105,106]. The patients were randomized to receive placebo or methotrexate at doses ranging from 7.5 to 20 mg per week plus corticosteroids. Both studies found little difference between the methotrexate groups and the placebo groups. There were no statistically significant differences in total steroid doses and steroid-related side effects.

Another randomized, placebo-controlled study of 42 patients showed some benefit to the addition of methotrexate [107]. In this study, patients were randomized to receive methotrexate 10 mg/wk or placebo in addition to a tapering prednisone dose starting at 60 mg/d. The researchers found 45% fewer relapses in the patients on methotrexate. This helped keep the total corticosteroid burden significantly lower in the methotrexate-treated patients. They did not find a difference in the steroid-related side effects between the two groups, and three patients on methotrexate had drug-related side effects. Although their findings are promising, the study may have been too small to suggest methotrexate treatment for all patients with GCA. This conflicting evidence makes is difficult to recommend the routine use of methotrexate in the treatment of GCA (grade of recommendation: D).

Other case reports or small studies have looked at the corticosteroid-sparing effects of a number of other medications. Etanercept and infliximab have promising case reports, but no formal studies have been done [108–110]. The results of a small placebo-controlled study with azathioprine are promising, but no significant follow-up studies have confirmed these findings [111]. Dapsone was studied and may be harmful [112]. The toxicity of long-term steroid treatment necessitates further research into steroid-sparing regimens.

The other aim in treatment of GCA has been to avoid the ischemic consequences. The effects of acetylsalicylic acid have been followed in a number studies investigating patients with GCA. A 2004 retrospective study found that patients who had been taking aspirin at low doses for cardiac reasons had a reduced rate of vision loss or stroke [113]. Only 8% of the patients taking aspirin had cranial ischemic events, compared with

29% of the patients not on aspirin. Another analysis of patients with CGA-related ischemic events also found that patients who were on aspirin had fewer events [114]. Although a randomized, controlled study of aspirin use has not been published, the use of aspirin in the prevention of CGA-related ischemia looks promising. The current recommendation is to start GCA patients on low-dose aspirin (grade of recommendation: B).

Prognosis

Although patients who present with strong inflammatory symptoms (eg, fever, weight loss, and anemia) and a highly elevated sedimentation rate rarely develop cranial ischemic complications [115], ischemic complications, particularly visual loss, cause the greatest morbidity in patients with GCA. Therefore, most of the prognostic research involves these problems. In one study of 185 patients with GCA, 41 patients had some visual loss [116]. This included involvement of 63 eyes causing vision loss to an acuity of <20/200 in 70% of effected eyes. Twenty-one percent of effected eyes had no light perception. Other studies have shown that treatment with various doses of corticosteroids has some minimal help in reversing vision loss. Late-onset permanent visual problems rarely occurred when GCA was treated before the development of vision loss [117].

Corticosteroid doses should be titrated for symptom resolution. Doses should be decreased if a patient is symptom free, but many patients have relapses of cranial symptoms. Doses should be up-titrated to resolve symptoms. Using laboratory values to direct titration of medication dose has not been proven to be helpful. Because GCA is a self-limited disease, most patients do not require life-long treatment with corticosteroids. A number of studies have found the average time on steroids to range from 24 to 30 months. Corticosteroid-induced side effects have been shown to cause morbidity in patients.

One of the most alarming findings in GCA arteritis is the high number of patients who develop aortic aneurysm and dissection. Aneurysm can develop after the initial diagnosis of GCA. Many of these patients develop aortic dissection and die. For this reason, screening for aortic aneurysm development recommendations in patients with GCA has been proposed. This includes a recommendation of life-long yearly imaging of the thoracic aorta with ultrasound or CT.

Although one study reported that older patients who experience total blindness have a higher short-term death rate [118], other studies have shown no difference in 5-year mortality. Five-year follow-up was obtained from 96% of the patients studied in the 1990 American College of Rheumatology classification study for GCA [24]. The researchers found that standard mortality rates were virtually identical in the GCA patients as in the general population.

Key Points

- PMR is a systemic inflammatory disease that occurs almost exclusively in patients older than 50 years of age.
- PMR is characterized by sudden onset, proximal extremity pain, morning stiffness, and rapid relief with the administration of corticosteroids.
- PMR occurs most frequently in Caucasians, particularly those of northern European descent, and is nearly two times more common in women.
- GCA is a vasculitic disease found in adults over 50 years of age, and the incidence increases with age.
- Classic symptoms of GCA include headache, scalp pain, visual disturbance, and jaw claudication. Some patients may present as fever of unknown origin.

References

[1] Salvarani C, Cantini F, Boiardi L, et al. Polymyalgia rheumatica and giant cell arteritis. N Engl J Med 2002;347:261–71.

[2] Weyand C, Goronzy J. Giant-cell arteritis and polymyalgia rheumatica. Ann Intern Med 2003;139:505–15.

[3] Meskimen S, Cook T, Blake R Jr. Management of giant cell arteritis and polymyalgia rheumatica. Am Fam Physician 2000;61:2061–8.

[4] Calvo-Romero JM. Giant cell arteritis. Postgrad Med J 2003;79:511–5.

[5] Nordberg E. Epidemiology of biopsy-positive giant cell arteritis: an overview. Clin Exp Rheum 2000;18(Suppl 20):S15–7.

[6] Doran M, Crowson CS, O'Fallon WM, et al. Trends in the incidence of polymyalgia rheumatica over a 30 year period in Olmstead County, Minnesota, USA. J Rheumatol 2002;29:1694–7.

[7] Salvarani C, Gabriel S, O'Fallon WM, et al. Epidemiology of polymyalgia rheumatica in Olmstead County, Minnesota, 1970–1991. Arthritis Rheum 1995;38:369–73.

[8] González-Gay MA, Garcia-Porrua C, Vazquez-Caruncho M, et al. The spectrum of polymyalgia rheumatica in Northwestern Spain: incidence and analysis of variables associated with relapse in a 10 year study. J Rheumatol 1999;26:1326–32.

[9] Cimmino MA, Caporali R, Montecucco CM, et al. A seasonal pattern in the onset of polymyalgia rheumatica. Ann Rheum Dis 1990;49:521–3.

[10] Duhaut P, Bosshard S, Calvet A, et al. Giant cell arteritis, polymyalgia rheumatica, and viral hypotheses: a multicenter, prospective case-control study. Groupe de Recherche sur l'Arterite a Cellules Geantes. J Rheumatol 1999;26:361–9.

[11] Duhaut P, Bosshard S, Dumontet C. Giant cell arteritis and polymyalgia rheumatica: role of viral infections. Clin Exp Rheumatol 2000;18(Suppl 20):S22–3.

[12] Elling P, Olsson AT, Elling H. Synchronous variations of the incidence of temporal arteritis and polymyalgia rheumatica in different regions of Denmark: association with epidemics of Mycoplasma pneumoniae infection. J Rheumatol 1996;23:112–9.

[13] Gabriel S, Espy M, Erdman D, et al. The role of parvovirus B19 in the pathogenesis of giant cell arteritis: a preliminary evaluation. Arthritis Rheum 1999;42:1255–8.

[14] Narváez J, Clavaguera MT, Nolla-Sole JM, et al. Lack of association between infection and onset of polymyalgia rheumatica. J Rheumatol 2000;27:953–7.

[15] Peris P. Polymyalgia rheumatica is not seasonal in pattern and is unrelated to parvovirus B19 infection. J Rheumatol 2003;30:2624–6.

[16] Hemauer A, Modrow S, Georgi J, et al. There is no association between polymyalgia rheumatica and acute parvovirus B19 infection. Ann Rheum Dis 1999;58:657–8.

[17] Roche N, Fulbright JW, Wagner AD, et al. Correlation of interleukin-6 production and disease activity in polymyalgia rheumatica and giant cell arteritis. Arthritis Rheum 1993;36:1286–94.

[18] Narváez J, Nolla-Solé J, Narváez JA, et al. Musculoskeletal manifestations in polymyalgia rheumatica and temporal cell arteritis. Ann Rheum Dis 2001;60:1060–3.

[19] Frediani B, Falsetti P, Storri L, et al. Evidence for synovitis in active polymyalgia rheumatica: sonographic study in a large series of patients. J Rheumatol 2002;29: 123–30.

[20] Cantini F, Salvarani C, Olivieri I, et al. Shoulder ultrasonography in the diagnosis of polymyalgia rheumatica: a case-control study. J Rheumatol 2001;28:1049–55.

[21] Salvarani C, Cantini F, Olivieri I, et al. Proximal bursitis in active polymyalgia rheumatica. Ann Intern Med 1997;127:27–31.

[22] Pavlica P, Barozzi L, Salvarani C, et al. Magnetic resonance imaging in the diagnosis of PMR. Clin Exp Rheumatol 2000;18(Suppl 20):S38–9.

[23] McGonagle D, Pease C, Marzo-Ortega H, et al. Comparison of extracapsular changes by magnetic resonance imaging in patients with rheumatoid arthritis and polymyalgia rheumatica. J Rheumatol 2001;28:1837–41.

[24] Matteson EL, Gold KN, Bloch DA, et al. Long-term survival of patients with giant cell arteritis in the American College of Rheumatology giant cell arteritis classification criteria cohort. Am J Med 1996;100:193–6.

[25] Salvarani C, Gabriel S, Hunder G. Distal extremity swelling with pitting edema in polymyalgia rheumatica. Arthritis Rheum 1996;39(1):73–80.

[26] Mandell B. Polymyalgia rheumatica: clinical presentation is key to diagnosis and treatment. Clev Clin J Med 2004;71:489–95.

[27] Östör A, Hazleman B. Managing the patient with polymyalgia. Practitioner 2002;246: 756–63.

[28] Chuang TY, Hunder GG, Ilstrup DM, et al. Polymyalgia rheumatica: a 10-year epidemiologic and clinical study. Ann Intern Med 1982;97:672–80.

[29] Healey LA. Polymyalgia rheumatica and the American Rheumatism Association criteria for rheumatoid arthritis. Arthritis Rheum 1983;26:1417–8.

[30] Lane SK, Gravel JW. Clinical utility of common serum rheumatologic tests. Am Fam Physician 2002;65:1073–80.

[31] Helfgott S, Kieval R. Polymyalgia rheumatica in patients with a normal erthrocyte sedimentation rate. Arthritis Rheum 1996;39(2):304–7.

[32] Gonzalez-Gay MA, Rodriguez-Valerde V, Blanca R, et al. Polymyalgia rheumatica without significantly increased erythrocyte sedimentation rate: a more benign syndrome. Arch Intern Med 1997;157:317–20.

[33] Cantini F, Salvarani C, Olivieri I, et al. Inflamed shoulder structures in polymyalgia rheumatica with normal erythrocyte sedimentation rate. Arthritis Rheum 2001;44: 1155–9.

[34] Miller J, Allen S, Walker S. Polymyalgia rheumatica. Available at: www.hypertension-consult.com/Secure/textbookarticles/Primary_Care_Book/148.htm. Accessed October 31, 2004.

[35] Weyand CM, Fulbright JW, Evans JM, et al. Corticosteroid requirements in polymyalgia rheumatica. Arch Intern Med 1999;159(6):577–84.

[36] Van der Veen MJ, Dintant HJ, van Booma-Frankfort C, et al. Can methotrexate be used as a steroid sparing agent in the treatment of polymyalgia rheumatica and giant cell arteritis? Ann Rheum Dis 1996;55:218–23.

[37] Caporali R, Cimmino MA, Ferraccioli G, et al. Prednisone plus methotrexate for polymyalgia rheumatica: a randomized, double-blind, placebo-controlled trial. Ann Intern Med 2004;141:493–500.

[38] Stone J. Methotrexate in polymyalgia rheumatica: kernel of truth or curse of Tantalus? [editorial] Ann Intern Med 2004;141:568–9.

[39] Lawrence RC, Helmick CG, Arnett FC, et al. Estimates of the prevalence of arthritis and selected musculoskeletal disorders in the United States. Arthritis Rheum 1998;41: 778–99.

[40] Salvarani C, Gabriel SE, O'Fallon WM, et al. The Incidence of giant cell arteritis in Olmstead County, Minnesota: apparent fluctuations in a cyclic pattern. Ann Intern Med 1995;123:192–4.

[41] Regan MJ, Wood BJ, Hsieh YH, et al. Temporal arteritis and chlamydia pneumoniae: failure to detect the organism by polymerase chain reaction in ninety cases and ninety controls. Arthritis Rheum 2002;46:1056–60.

[42] Bonnet F, Morlat P, Delevaux I, et al. A possible association between Chlamydiae psittaci infection and temporal arteritis. Joint Bone Spine 2000;67:550–2.

[43] Mitchell BM, Font RL. Detection of varicella zoster virus DNA in some patients with giant cell arteritis. Invest Ophthalmol Vis Sci 2001;42:2572–7.

[44] Hunder GG. Pathogenesis of giant cell (temporal) arteritis. UpToDate 2004;12(2): 1–7.

[45] Cid MC, Hernandez-Rodriguez J, Esteban MJ, et al. Tissue and serum angiogenic activity is associated with low prevalence of ischemic complications in patients with giant-cell arteritis. Circulation 2002;106:1664–71.

[46] Calamia KT, Hunder GG. Giant cell arteritis (temporal arteritis) presenting as fever of undetermined origin. Arthritis Rheum 1981;24:1414–8.

[47] Liozon E, Boutros-Toni F, Ly K, et al. Silent, or masked, giant cell arteritis is associated with a strong inflammatory response and a benign short term course. J Rheum 2003;30: 1272–6.

[48] Gonzalez-Gay MA, Garcia-Porrua C, Amor-Dorado JC, et al. Fever in biopsy-proven giant cell arteritis: clinical implication in a defined population. Arthritis Rheum 2004;51: 652–5.

[49] Myklebust G, Gran JT. A prospective study of 287 patients with polymyalgia rheumatica and temporal arteritis: clinical and laboratory manifestations at onset of disease and at the time of diagnosis. Br J Rheum 1996;35:1161–8.

[50] Hunder GG. Clinical manifestations and diagnosis of giant cell (temporal arteritis). UpToDate 2004;12(2):1–16.

[51] Hunder GG, Bloch DA, Michel BA, et al. The American College of Rheumatology 1990 criteria for the classification of giant cell arteritis. Arthritis Rheum 1990;33: 1122–9.

[52] Cikes A, Depairon M, Joidon RM, et al. Necrosis of the tongue and unilateral blindness in temporal arteritis. Vasa 2001;30:222–4.

[53] Nir-Paz R, Gross A, Chojek-Shaul T. Reduction of jaw opening (trismus) in giant cell arteritis. Ann Rheum Dis 2002;61:832–3.

[54] Liozon E, Jauberteau MO, Ly K, et al. Reduction in jaw opening in giant cell arteritis. Ann Rheum Dis 2003;62:287–8.

[55] Ruiz-Masera JJ, Alamillos-Grandos FJ, Dean-Ferrer A, et al. Submandibular swelling as the first manifestation of giant cell arteritis: report of a case. J Cranio-Maxillo-Facial Surg 1995;23:119–21.

[56] Gordon LK, Levin LA. Visual loss in giant cell arteritis. JAMA 1998;280:385–6.

[57] Aiello PD, Trautman JC, McPhee TJ, et al. Visual prognosis in giant cell arteritis. Ophthalmology 1993;100:550–5.

[58] Font C, Cid MC, Coll-Vinent B, et al. Clinical features in patients with permanent visual loss due to biopsy-proven giant cell arteritis. Br J Rheum 1997;36:251–4.

[59] Nuenninghoff DM, Hunder GG, Christianson TJ, et al. Incidence and predictors of large-artery complication (aortic aneurysm, aortic dissection, and/or large artery stenosis) in patients with giant cell arteritis: a population-based study over 50 years. Arthritis Rheum 2003;48:3522–31.

[60] Brack A, Martinez-Taboada V, Stanson A, et al. Disease pattern in cranial and large-vessel giant cell arteritis. Arthritis Rheum 1999;42:311–7.

[61] Evans JM, O'Fallon WM, Hunder GG. Increased incidence of aortic aneurysm and dissection in giant cell (temporal) arteritis: a population-based study. Ann Intern Med 1995;122:505–7.

[62] Gonzalez-Gay MA, Blanco R, Rodriguez-Valverde V, et al. Permanent visual loss and cerebrovascular accidents in giant cell arteritis: predictors and response to treatment. Arthritis Rheum 1998;41:1497–504.

[63] Uddhammar A, Eriksson AL, Nystrom L, et al. Increased mortality due to cardiovascular disease in patients with giant cell arteritis in northern Sweden J Rheum 2002;29:737–42.

[64] Anim JT, van Herk EJ. Giant cell arteritis of the breast. Med Princ Pract 2004;13: 234–6.

[65] Burton EA, Winer JB, Barber PC. Giant cell arteritis of the cervical radicular vessels presenting with diaphragmatic weakness. J Neurol Neurosurg Psychiatry 1999;67: 223–6.

[66] Amor-Dorado JC, Llorca J, Costa-Ribas C, et al. Giant cell arteritis: a new association with benign paroxysmal positional vertigo. Laryngoscope 2004;114:1420–5.

[67] Miller A, Green M, Robinson D. Simple rule for calculating normal erythrocyte sedimentation rate. BMJ 1983;286:266.

[68] Smentana GW, Shmerling RH. Does this patient have temporal arteritis? JAMA 2002;287: 92–101.

[69] Salvarani C, Hunder GG. Giant cell arteritis with low erythrocyte sedimentation rate: frequency of occurrence in a population-based study. Arthritis Rheum 2001;45: 140–5.

[70] Kyle V, Cawston TE, Hazleman BL. Erythrocyte sedimentation rate and C reactive protein in the assessment of polymyalgia rheumatica: giant cell arteritis on presentation and during follow up. Ann Rheum Dis 1989;48:667–71.

[71] Eshaghian J, Goeken JA. C-reactive protein in giant cell (crania, temporal) arteritis. Ophthalmology 1980;87:1160–6.

[72] Costello F, Zimmerman MB, Podhajsky PA, et al. Role of thrombocytosis in the diagnosis of giant cell arteritis and differentiation of arteric from non-arteric anterior ischemic optic neuropathy. Eur J Ophthalmol 2004;14:245–57.

[73] Foroozan R, Danesh-Meyer H, Savino PJ, et al. Thrombocytosis in patients with biopsy-proven giant cell arteritis. Ophthalmology 2002;109:1267–71.

[74] Lincoff NS, Erlich PD, Brass LS. Thrombocytosis in temporal arteritis rising platelet counts: a red flag for giant cell arteritis. J Neuro-Ophthalmol 2000;20:67–72.

[75] Mana R, Cristiano G, Todaro L, et al. Microscopic hematuria: a diagnostic aid in giant cell arteritis. Lancet 1997;350:1226.

[76] Liozon E, Roblot P, Paire D, et al. Anticardiolipin antibody levels predict flares and relapses in patients with giant-cell (temporal) arteritis: a longitudinal study of 58 biopsy-proven cases. J Rheum 2000;39:1089–94.

[77] Walz LeBlanc BA, Keystone EC, Feltis JT, et al. Polyarteritis nodosa clinically masquerading as temporal arteritis with lymphadenopathy. J Rheum 1994;21:949–52.

[78] Younge BR, Cook BE, Bartley GB, et al. Initiation of glucocorticoid therapy: before or after temporal artery biopsy? Mayo Clin Proc 2004;79:483–91.

[79] Rodriguez-Valverde V, Sarabria JM, Gonzalez-Gay MA, et al. Risk factors and predictive models of giant cell arteritis in polymyalgia rheumatica. Am J Med 1997;102:331–6.

[80] Gabriel SE, O'Fallon WM, Achkar AA, et al. The use of clinical characteristics to predict the results of temporal artery biopsy among patients with suspected giant cell arteritis. J Rheum 1995;22:93–6.

[81] Schmidt WA, Kraft HE, Vorpahl K, et al. Color duplex ultrasound in the diagnosis of temporal arteritis. New Engl J Med 1997;337:1336–42.

[82] Salvarani C, Mauro S, Angelo G, et al. Is duplex ultrasonography useful for the diagnosis of giant-cell arteritis? Ann Intern Med 2002;137:232–8.

[83] Lesar CJ, Meier GH, DeMasi RJ, et al. The utility of color duplex ultrasound in the diagnosis of temporal arteritis. J Vasc Surg 2002;36:1154–60.

[84] Pfadenhauer K, Weber H. Duplex sonography of temporal and occipital artery in the diagnosis of temporal arteritis: a prospective study. J Rheum 2003;30:2177–81.

[85] Pfadenhauer K, Weber H. Giant cell arteritis of the occipital arteries: a prospective color coded duplex sonography study in 78 patients. J Neurol 2003;250:844–9.

[86] Turlakow A, Yeung HW, Pui J, et al. Fludeoxyglucose positron emission tomography in the diagnosis of giant cell arteritis. Arch Intern Med 2001;161:1003–7.

[87] Brodmann M, Lipp RW, Passath A, et al. The role of 2-18F-fluoro-2-deoxy-D-glucose positron emission tomography in the diagnosis of giant cell arteritis on the temporal arteries. J Rheum 2004;43:241–2.

[88] Genereau T, Lortholary O, Guillevin L, et al. Temporal 67 gallium uptake is increase in temporal arteritis. J Rheum 1999;38:709–13.

[89] Reitblat T, Ben-Horin CL, Reitblat A. Gallium-67 SPECT scintigraphy may be useful in diagnosis of temporal arteritis. Ann Rheum Dis 2003;62:257–60.

[90] Kent RB, Thomas L. Temporal artery biopsy. Am Surg 1990;56:16–21.

[91] Hall S, Lie JT, Kurland LT, et al. The therapeutic impact of temporal artery biopsy. Lancet 1983;2:1217–20.

[92] Sudlow C. Diagnosing and managing polymyalgia rheumatica and temporal arteritis: sensitivity of temporal artery biopsy varies with biopsy length and sectioning strategy. BMJ 1997;315:549.

[93] Danesh-Meyer HV, Savino PJ, Eagle RC, et al. Low diagnostic yield with second biopsy in suspected giant cell arteritis. J Neuro-Ophthalmol 2000;20:213–5.

[94] Hall JK, Volpe NJ, Galetta SL, et al. The role of unilateral temporal artery biopsy. Ophthalmology 2003;110:543–8.

[95] Achkar AA, Lie JT, Hunder GG, et al. How does previous corticosteroid treatment affect the biopsy findings in giant cell (temporal) arteritis? Ann Intern Med 1994;120: 987–92.

[96] Ray-Chaudhuri N, Kine DA, Tijani SO, et al. Effects of prior steroid treatment on temporal artery biopsy findings in giant cell arteritis. Br J Ophthalmol 2002;86:530–2.

[97] Chan CCK, Paine M, O'Day J. Steroid management in giant cell arteritis. Br J Ophthalmol 2001;85:1061–4.

[98] Foroozan R, Deramo VA, Buono LM, et al. Recovery of visual function in patients with biopsy-proven giant cell arteritis. Ophthalmology 2003;110:539–42.

[99] Chevalet P, Barrier JH, Pottier P, et al. A randomized, multicenter, controlled trial using intravenous pulses of methylprednisolone in the initial treatment of simple forms of giant cell arteritis: a one year followup study of 164 patients. J Rheum 2000;27:1484–91.

[100] Delecoeuillerie G, Joly P, Cohen de Lara A, et al. Polymyalgia rheumatica and temporal arteritis: a retrospective analysis of prognostic features and different corticosteroid regimens (11 year survey of 210 patients). Ann Rheum Dis 1988;47:733–9.

[101] Lundberg I, Hedfors E. Restricted dose and duration of corticosteroid treatment in patients with polymyalgia rheumatica and temporal arteritis. J Rheum 1990;17:1340–5.

[102] Myles AB, Perera T, Ridley MG. Prevention of blindness in giant cell arteritis by corticosteroid treatment. Br J Rheum 1992;31:103–5.

[103] Myklebust G, Gran JT. Prednisolone maintenance dose in relation to starting dose in the treatment of polymyalgia rheumatica and temporal arteritis: a prospective two-year study of 273 patients. Scand J Rheum 2001;30:260–7.

[104] Kyle V, Hazleman BL. Treatment of polymyalgia rheumatica and giant cell arteritis: I. Steroid regimens in the first two months. Ann Rheum Dis 1989;48:658–61.

[105] Spiera RF, Mitnick HJ, Kupersmith M, et al. A prospective, double-blind, randomized placebo controlled trial of methotrexate in the treatment of giant cell arteritis. Clin Exp Rheumatol 2001;19:495–501.

[106] Hoffman GS, Cid MC, Hellmann DB, et al. A multicenter, randomized, double-blind, placebo-controlled trial of adjuvant methotrexate treatment for giant cell arteritis. Arthritis Rheum 2002;46:1309–18.

[107] Jover JA, Hernandez-Garcia C, Morado IC, et al. Combined treatment of giant-cell arteritis with methotrexate and prednisone. Ann Intern Med 2001;134:106–14.

[108] Tan AL, Holdworth J, Pease C, et al. Successful treatment of resistant giant cell arteritis with etanercept. Ann Rheum Dis 2003;62:373–4.

[109] Cantini F, Niccoli L, Slavarani C, et al. Treatment of longstanding active giant cell arteritis with infliximab: report of four cases. Arthritis Rheum 2001;44:2933–5.

[110] Airo P, Antonioli CM, Vianelli M, et al. Anti-tumor necrosis factor treatment with infliximab in a case of giant cell arteritis resistant to steroid and immunosuppressive drugs. Rheum 2002;41:347–9.

[111] De Silva M, Hazleman BL. Azathioprine in giant cell arteritis/polymyalgia rheumatica: a double blind study. Ann Rheum Dis 1986;45:136–8.

[112] Liozon F, Vidal E, Barrier JH. Dapsone in giant cell arteritis treatment. Eur J Int Med 1993;4:207–14.

[113] Nesher G, Berkun Y, Mates M, et al. Low-dose aspirin and prevention of cranial ischemic complications in giant cell arteritis. Arthritis Rheum 2004;50:1332–7.

[114] Nesher G, Berkun Y, Mates M, et al. Risk factors for cranial ischemic complications in giant cell arteritis. Medicine 2004;83:114–22.

[115] Cid MC, Font C, Oristrell J, et al. Association between strong inflammatory response and low risk of developing visual loss and other cranial ischemic complications in giant cell (temporal) arteritis. Arthritis Rheum 1998;41:26–32.

[116] Liu GT, Glaser JS, Schatz NJ, et al. Visual morbidity in giant cell arteritis: Clinical characteristics and prognosis for vision. Ophthalmology 1994;101:1779–85.

[117] Kupersmith MJ, Langer R, Mitnick H, et al. Visual performance in giant cell arteritis (temporal arteritis) after 1 year of therapy. Br J Ophthalmol 1999;83:796–801.

[118] Liozon E, Loustaud-Ratti V, Ly K, et al. Visual prognosis in extremely old patients with temporal (giant cell) arteritis. J Am Geriatr Soc 2003;51:722–3.

Address reprint requests to

John Donnelly, MD
200 Hygeia Drive
Newark, DE 19713

e-mail: jdonnelly@christianacare.org

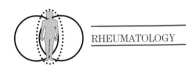 RHEUMATOLOGY 1522–5720/05 $15.00 + .00

COMMON SPORTS INJURIES: UPPER EXTREMITY INJURIES

Rajwinder S. Deu, MD, and Peter J. Carek, MD, MS

Injuries are common in athletics, with factors such as overuse, misuse, and underlying disease as causes. Many injuries are the product of a single-event macrotrauma (acute injuries), single-event trauma to tissue made vulnerable by overuse (acute on chronic), or multiple-repetition overuse (chronic) [1]. Overuse injuries make up the most common subtype affecting athletes, resulting from repetitive microtrauma leading to inflammation and local tissue damage. Intrinsic and extrinsic factors contribute to the overload that causes overuse injuries. Intrinsic refers to natural biomechanical abnormalities, such as malalignments, muscle imbalance, inflexibility, weakness, and instability [2,3]. Extrinsic (ie, avoidable) factors include poor technique, improper equipment, and improper changes in the duration or frequency of activity [2,3]. A majority of these individuals present to their primary care physician for initial evaluation. The primary care physician must have understanding and knowledge of these disorders so that proper care can be given.

Common injuries of the upper extremity include trigger finger, De Quervain tenosynovitis, mallet finger, carpal tunnel syndrome, lateral epicondylitis, olecranon bursitis, and rotator cuff tendinitis.

TRIGGER FINGER

Clinical Presentation

Stenosing tenosynovitis, or "trigger finger," is a condition involving the flexor tendon of the thumb or individual finger causing catching or locking

From the Department of Family Medicine, Thomas Jefferson University, Philadelphia, Pennsylvania; the Trident/MUSC Family Medicine Residency Program, Medical University of South Carolina, Charleston, South Carolina; and the Department of Family Medicine, Medical University of South Carolina, Charleston, South Carolina of the digit in flexion. Patients often report pain located at the proximal interphalangeal (PIP) joint of the finger or the interphalangeal (IP) joint of the thumb. Trigger finger is the most common entrapment tendonitis in the hand and wrist [4]. Trigger Finger is found more commonly in women, with a frequency 2 to 6 times that observed in men. It usually presents in the fifth and sixth decades of life [5]. The thumb is most frequently involved, followed by the fourth and middle fingers.

Triggering is usually localized to the region of the first annular (A1) pulley of the flexor tendon sheath. Specifically, localized swelling of the flexor digitorum superficialis interferes with the normal gliding mechanism, causing the tendon to get caught under the A1 pulley at the metacarpophalangeal (MP) joint. This thickening may develop into a nodule on the tendon, causing the tendon to stick at the proximal edge of the A1 pulley and locking the finger in flexion. The individual suffering from trigger finger commonly needs to apply an external force on the digit to obtain complete extension.

Physical Examination

The examiner may observe the affected digit locked in a flexed position and then snap or trigger when it is forcefully extended. The patient commonly complains of pain at the PIP or IP joint. Palpation of the MP joint over the palmar crease reveals a tender nodule that moves with flexion and extension of the finger.

Diagnostic Studies

Unless a fracture is suspected, no imaging studies are needed in cases of trigger finger.

Treatment

Initial treatment is aimed toward the inflammation surrounding the tendon. Activity modification, nonsteroidal anti-inflammatory drugs (NSAIDs), splinting, and local steroid injection into the tendon sheath are initial treatment options. Activity modification includes minimizing activities that involve repetitive and prolonged gripping and grasping (grade of recommendation: D) (Table 1). A hand-based splint that prevents motion of the MP and PIP/IP joints may be worn at night to prevent excessive flexing and locking during sleep (grade of recommendation: C). Caution should be used with the amount of time spent in the splint to avoid permanent stiffness. Patel et al [6] found that 66% of patients with their MP joint splinted at 10° to 15° of flexion for 6 weeks had relief of symptoms [6]. Many clinicians offer corticosteroid injection at the area of thickening in

TABLE 1.
Grades of Recommendation for Selected Treatments

Condition	Treatment	Grade of Recommendation
Trigger finger	Activity modification	D
	NSAIDs	D
	Splinting	C
	Corticosteroid injection	C
De Quervain tenosynovitis	Activity modification	Not recommended
	NSAIDs	Not recommended
	Splinting	C
	Corticosteroid injection	C
Mallet finger	Splinting	C
Carpal tunnel syndrome	Activity modification	D
	Ergonomic keyboards	D
	Splinting	B
	NSAIDs	Not recommended
	Vitamin B6	Not recommended
	Oral corticosteroid	A
	Corticosteroid injection	A
Lateral epicondylitis	Activity modification	D
	Oral NSAIDs	B
	Topical NSAIDs	B
	Physical therapy	A
	Counterforce bracing	D
	Corticosteroid injection	A
	Extracorporeal shock wave therapy	D
	Acupuncture	D
Olecranon bursitis	Ice	D
	NSAIDs	D
	Compression	D
	Aspiration	D
	Corticosteroid injection	D
Rotator cuff tendinitis	Physical therapy	C
	Subacromial corticosteroid injection	D

Abbreviation: NSAID, nonsteroidal anti-inflammatory drug.

the tendon sheath as first-line therapy (grade of recommendation: C). The first injection has been found to relieve symptoms in roughly 84% of trigger fingers and in 92% of trigger thumbs, whereas a second injection increased relief to 91% and 97% of patients, respectively [6,7]. This injection can be repeated at 3-week intervals for a total of three injections [8]. The corticosteroid should not be injected directly into the tendon; this may cause tendon rupture. If three injections fail to provide adequate relief, then the patient should be referred for surgery. Surgical treatment involves percutaneous or open release of the A1 pulley.

DE QUERVAIN TENOSYNOVITIS

Clinical Presentation

De Quervain tenosynovitis is a stenosing tenosynovitis of the first dorsal compartment of the wrist, involving the abductor pollicis longus (APL) and extensor pollicis brevis (EPB). It is second to trigger finger as the most common entrapment tendonitis, occurring approximately one twentieth as often [4]. Patients complain of pain and tenderness localized to the dorsoradial aspect of the wrist that is exacerbated with thumb and wrist motion. De Quervain tenosynovitis occurs most commonly in women between 30 and 50 years of age [9]. Mothers of infants aged 6 to 12 months and day care workers are frequently affected due to repetitive lifting of infants.

In De Quervain tenosynovitis, the tendons of the APL and EPB become thickened from acute or repetitive trauma and interfere with the normal gliding mechanism through the sheath. Continued thumb motion, along with radial and ulnar deviation of the wrist, perpetuates the inflammation and swelling.

Physical Examination

The first dorsal compartment over the radial styloid is thickened and tender to palpation. Crepitus may be felt on active and passive thumb motion. Finkelstein's test is positive, causing sharp pain over the first dorsal compartment. This maneuver is done by having the patient flex the thumb into the palm and then make a fist. The wrist is passively deviated in the ulnar direction, which places stress on the APL and EPB. Axial loading of the carpometacarpal (CMC) joint should be performed to rule out arthritis at the joint.

Diagnostic Studies

Radiographs are not necessary for diagnosis, although they may be helpful to rule out other conditions that may be responsible, such as CMC joint arthritis.

Treatment

Initial treatment attempts to decrease the inflammation surrounding the tendons. Activity modification, NSAIDs, splinting, and local steroid injection into the tendon sheath are common treatment options. A pooled quantitative literature evaluation found no benefit for rest or NSAID use (not recommended) [10]. Splinting involves immobilization of the thumb and wrist in a partially flexed position (grade of recommendation: C). It has been found to provide complete relief in 14% to 19% of patients [10,11]. Injection of the tendon sheath of the first distal compartment reduces tendon thickening and inflammation and provides the most effective form of treatment (grade of recommendation: C). The first injection has been found to relieve symptoms in roughly 66% to 70% of patients, and a second injection permanently relieves symptoms in another 10% of patients [11,12]. Use of injections along with splinting has been less effective, providing relief in 57% to 62% of patients [10,11,13]. The duration of symptoms before treatment does not seem to affect the outcome [12,13]. Patients who fail injection therapy should be referred for surgical release of the first dorsal compartment.

MALLET FINGER

Clinical Presentation

Mallet finger, also known as "baseball finger" or "drop finger," involves disruption of the extensor tendon or an avulsion fracture of the distal phalanx. This injury occurs with a forced flexion against an actively extended distal interphalangeal (DIP) joint resulting in a characteristic flexion deformity or drooping of the DIP joint. The classic mechanism involves a direct blow to the tip of the finger while the DIP joint is held in extension. Although this injury is commonly caused during participation in athletic activities (eg, by contact with a baseball, volleyball, or basketball), mallet finger may occur with household activities, such as pushing off a sock or tucking in bedsheets.

Physical Examination

With mallet finger, a flexion deformity at the DIP joint with the patient unable to actively extend the distal phalanx is present. Swelling and tenderness may be found on the dorsum of the joint. Commonly, the injury is painless, causing patients to wait weeks to months before being seen and therefore causing patients to present with a subsequent swan neck deformity. A swan neck deformity is caused by the unopposed extensor mechanism on the middle phalanx leading to hyperextension of the PIP joint.

Diagnostic Studies

Radiographs (Posterioanterior, lateral, and oblique centered at the DIP joint) are used to differentiate between an injury to the bone or tendon.

The lateral view allows for visualization of a bony avulsion at the dorsal base of the distal phalanx.

Treatment

Treatment of mallet finger consists of continuous splinting of the DIP joint in full extension or slight hyperextension. Splinting must be done for a minimum of 6 weeks; tendon injuries require up to 8 weeks. After the initial period, night splinting is conducted for 2 weeks, and splinting is continued during athletic activities for an additional 4 weeks. The key to treatment is continuous splinting because any flexion of the DIP joint before the prescribed treatment time can lead to reinjury.

Surgery is recommended for displaced avulsion fractures with a large articular component (more than 50% of the joint surface), volar subluxation of the distal phalanx, or failure of splinting.

A Cochrane review looking at interventions for treating mallet finger injuries found insufficient evidence to establish the effectiveness of different finger splints in determining when surgery is indicated (grade of recommendation: D). The review did find that patient adherence to splint use was important (grade of recommendation: C) [14].

CARPAL TUNNEL SYNDROME

Clinical Presentation

Carpal tunnel syndrome (CTS) results from compression of the median nerve at the wrist. Patients complain of pain, numbness, and tingling in the distribution of the median nerve, although all fingers are commonly involved. Because patients may flex the wrist while sleeping, symptoms are usually worse at night and commonly awaken patients. Individuals occasionally complain of decreased grip strength causing them to drop objects.

CTS is the most common peripheral nerve compression syndrome. The estimated lifetime risk of acquiring CTS is 10%; there is an annual incidence of 50 to 150 cases per 100,000 population and an overall prevalence between 2.7% to 3% [15–17]. CTS typically occurs after 30 years of age and is three times more common in women than in men [15,18].

Most cases of CTS are idiopathic. Common in people who perform repetitive motions of the hand and wrist, CTS can be caused by any injury or trauma to the area that causes swelling of the tissues within the carpal tunnel. Sports such as racquetball and handball or activities such as typing, driving, assembly-line work, and using vibratory tools (eg, jackhammers) are frequently associated with CTS. CTS has also been associated with a number of systemic conditions, including rheumatoid arthritis, diabetes, hypothyroidism, acromegaly, gout, renal failure, obesity, pregnancy, and menopause.

Physical Examination

The principal clinical tests for CTS are the provocative tests: Phalen's maneuver, Tinel's sign, and carpal compression test. Phalen's maneuver (sensitivity 67.5% to 72%, specificity 53% to 91%) consists of flexion of the wrist at 90° for 60 seconds [19,20]. For Tinel's sign (sensitivity 55% to 67.5%, specificity 72% to 90%), the examiner taps over the carpal tunnel [19,20]. The carpal compression test involves the application of direct pressure on the carpal canal with both thumbs of the examiner for 30 seconds. These tests are considered positive if symptoms (eg, paresthesias) develop in the median nerve distribution. Visual inspection of the hand may show thenar atrophy, and the patient may have weakness of resisted thumb abduction.

Diagnostic Tests

The diagnosis of CTS is challenging. Physical examination signs are only moderately sensitive. When the diagnosis or possible need for surgical intervention is in question, electrophysiology can be used for confirmation. The two tests commonly performed include nerve conduction velocity (NCV) and electromyography (EMG).

NCV measures the speed of conduction of impulses through the nerve by stimulating surface electrodes on the skin. In suspected CTS, a sensory latency of >3.5 milliseconds or a motor latency of >4.5 milliseconds is considered abnormal [21]. EMG assesses the health of muscles by measuring their electrical activity. Persons with CTS have sharp waves, fibrillation potentials, and increased insertional activity [21].

Even though nerve conduction studies are considered the standard for diagnosis, a number of patients suspected of having clinical CTS have normal results. Jablecki et al [22] compared pooled sensitivities and specificities of electrodiagnostic technique to diagnose CTS and found sensitivity of 0.56 to 0.85 and specificity of 0.94 to 0.99 [22]. In addition, no morphologic information regarding the median nerve and possible etiologic factors is provided by these studies. As a result, various other modalities, including ultrasound and MRI, have been investigated as alternatives.

Diagnostic ultrasound provides a noninvasive and cost-effective way of evaluating for CTS. El Miedany [23] and Kele [24] found a correlation between conduction abnormalities of the median nerve by electro-diagnostic tests and cross-sectional area of the nerve by ultrasound (P <0.05). Both studies found that ultrasound aided in defining the cause of nerve compression and suggested a specific therapeutic strategy.

MRI has been used in the diagnosis of CTS in individuals with ambiguous nerve conduction studies and clinical examinations. It is helpful in identifying normal carpal tunnel anatomy and pathologic nerve compression and mass lesions, such as ganglion cysts [25]. Mesgarzadeh et al [26] found that patients with CTS had swelling of the median nerve, flattening of the median nerve, palmar bowing of the flexor retinaculum, and increased signal intensity of the median nerve on T2-weighted images regardless of the cause of CTS. Radack et al [27] found high specificity for retinacular bowing (94%), median nerve flattening (97%), and deep palmar bursitis (95%).

Treatment

Various treatment modalities exist for CTS; treatment depends on severity of the disease. Mild to moderate disease can be treated non-operatively. Avoidance of repetitive wrist and hand motions that exacerbate symptoms, implementation of ergonomic measures, use of a wrist splint, oral medications, and local corticosteroid injection are initial treatment options.

Activity modification including avoidance of repetitive wrist and hand motions should be attempted initially. Vibratory tools (eg, jackhammers) should not be used because they may exacerbate symptoms (grade of recommendation: D). Implementing ergonomic measures for individuals who work on computers may help with wrist position to minimize stressful motions, although a Cochrane review comparing ergonomic keyboards versus control demonstrated equivocal results for pain and function (grade of recommendation: D) [28]. Activity modification can be aided with the use of splinting the wrist at a neutral angle to prevent repetitive flexion and rotation. Limited evidence supports a positive short-term effect on symptoms after the use of a hand splint for 2 or 3 weeks (grade of recommendation: B) [28]. Goodyear-Smith et al [15] performed a systematic review and found that splinting at night was not as effective as full-time splinting day and night [15]. Nightly splint use is usually recommended to prevent prolonged wrist flexion and extension because full-time splinting is felt to hinder daily activities.

Many medications have been used to treat CTS with varying results. A Cochrane review [28] and a systematic review performed by Gerritsen et al [29] concluded that diuretics, NSAIDs, and vitamin B6 offer no benefit. Corticosteroids, orally and by local injection, have been found to be beneficial for short-term relief [15]. Two-week oral steroid treatment compared with placebo demonstrated a significant improvement in symptoms [28]. Local steroid injection provided greater clinical improvement at 1 month compared with placebo [29,30]. Local corticosteroid injection provides significantly greater clinical improvement than oral steroid for up to 3 months after treatment (grade of recommendation: A) [30,31].

CTS is a progressive disease, and many patients eventually need surgery. Surgery should be considered for patients who fail non-operative treatment, for patients with severe nerve entrapment, or for patients with deterioration on nerve conduction studies. Surgery relieves symptoms significantly more than splinting [32]. Carpal tunnel release can be performed as an open procedure or endoscopically; patients improve significantly with either procedure [15]. Endoscopic procedure is thought to allow for earlier return to work or activities of daily living. However, a Cochrane review found no evidence to suggest the benefit of one procedure compared with the other [33].

LATERAL EPICONDYLITIS

Clinical Presentation

Lateral epicondylitis, also known as "tennis elbow," describes a condition involving the common extensor origin at the elbow. Patients complain primarily of pain located over the lateral aspect of the elbow triggered by wrist extension.

Lateral epicondylitis has been incorrectly termed a "tendonitis" due to the theory that inflammatory changes exist within the tendon. Histologic examination of affected tendons has failed to show inflammatory cells [34]. As a result, the term "tendinosis" is used instead, with the characteristic appearance of a tendon that is dull, gray, friable, and often edematous [34].

Pathogenesis of lateral epicondylitis has been linked with repetitive activities that require forceful wrist extension. Specifically, this repetitive motion results in changes within the proximal musculotendinous origin of the extensor carpi radialis brevis [35]. Even though this condition is commonly linked with tennis, only 5% to 10% of patients are tennis players [36]. Lateral epicondylitis is found in athletes who participate in baseball, golf, fencing, swimming, and track and field events that involve throwing [36,37]. The onset of symptoms usually occurs between 35 and 50 years of age, with a median age of 41 years, although it has been identified in patients ranging from 12 to 80 years of age [34]. No difference in prevalence between men and women has been noted, and this condition typically involves the dominant arm [36,38,39].

Numerous other etiologies responsible for lateral elbow pain exist and must be included in the differential diagnosis. Posterior interosseous nerve entrapment, C6-C7 cervical nerve root compression, synovitis, chondromalacia, bursitis, olecranon osteophytes, or radiocapitellar osteoarthritis are possible etiologies for lateral elbow pain [34,35].

Physical Examination

Patients complain of pain with palpation just distal to the lateral epicondyle over the extensor tendon location. Pain is reproduced with gripping, resisted wrist extension, resisted long finger extension, and resisted forearm supination. Decreased grip strength is noted with handgrip dynamometer, and range of motion can be decreased with loss of terminal extension in more chronic conditions.

Diagnostic Studies

Clinicians may use radiographic evaluation to rule out other pathologic conditions such as fracture, dislocation, degenerative changes, or loose bodies. This includes anterior-posterior (AP), lateral, and axial views of the elbow. Up to 20% of patients demonstrate tendon calcification or reactive exostosis of the epicondyle [34].

Ultrasound has proven to be a useful and inexpensive method to identify lateral epicondylitis. Affected tendons appear swollen and abnormally hypoechoic. Cortical irregularity can be seen on the epicondyle, and pain can be reproduced with transducer pressure [40]. Other studies, such as MRI, bone scan, and EMG, can be used to rule out etiologies such as posterior interosseous nerve entrapment and C6-C7 cervical nerve root compression.

Treatment

Various treatment modalities exist for lateral epicondylitis. Nirschl et al [34] found that approximately 95% of patients improve with conservative therapy. Initially, treatment includes modification of activity to avoid offending activities, such as limiting racquet use for tennis players or limiting repetitive stressors to laborers by changing job tasks or placing weight restrictions on their activities (grade of recommendation: D). Ice and NSAIDs may be helpful with acute onset of symptoms. A review found limited evidence of a short-term improvement in pain and function with an oral NSAID versus placebo, but NSAID use significantly reduces pain at 26 weeks (grade of recommendation: B) [41]. In addition, topical NSAIDs were found to significantly improve pain in the short term when compared with placebo (grade of recommendation: B) [41].

A physical therapy program that includes passive and active range of motion exercises and advancing to active and isometric resistance exercises may provide additional benefit [35]. Smidt et al [42] showed 91% success rate in patients who were treated with physiotherapy when measured at 52 weeks (grade of recommendation: A). A Cochrane review was unable to show a consistent benefit of deep-tendon friction massage combined with other physiotherapy modalities on control of pain, improvement of grip strength, or functional status [43].

Counterforce bracing may be used to decrease symptoms by limiting full contractile expansion of the musculotendinous unit that dissipates muscle contractile tension and distributes forces to nondiseased tissue [35,36]. A Cochrane review on use of orthotic devices in the treatment of tennis elbow was unable to draw any definitive conclusions on their effectiveness (grade of recommendation: D) [44].

Patients who do not respond to initial therapeutic measures may benefit from a local corticosteroid injection (grade of recommendation: A). Subcutaneous injection needs to be avoided because atrophy of the subcutaneous fatty tissue and skin depigmentation may occur. In a systematic review of randomized clinical trials, corticosteroid injections for lateral epicondylitis seem to be effective for short-term improvement in symptoms (2–6 weeks) [45]. Smidt et al [42] showed that corticosteroid injection had a 92% success rate at 6 weeks when compared with physiotherapy (47%) and wait-and-see (32%). Corticosteroid injection was found to provide less long-term relief at 52 weeks compared with the other outcome measures.

Numerous other treatment modalities, such as extracorporeal shock wave therapy (ESWT), acupuncture, ultrasonography, and percutaneous needling, have been attempted, but evidence for their benefit is lacking. Cochrane reviews looking at ESWT and acupuncture found insufficient data to support or refute their use (grade of recommendation: D) [46,47].

Individuals who fail to improve after completion of a non-operative treatment program, who report continued pain and disruption in quality of life, or who have symptoms that last from 6 to 12 months may benefit from surgery. Nirschl et al [34] have found that 85% of patients experienced full pain relief and full strength of return, 12% improved with some pain with strenuous activity, and 3% had no improvement. No evidence exists regarding trials of surgery for lateral elbow pain, which makes it difficult to make any conclusions on its value (grade of recommendation: D) [48].

OLECRANON BURSITIS

Clinical Presentation

Olecranon bursitis is an inflammation of the bursa that lies between the olecranon process and the overlying skin. This bursa acts to reduce friction and allow for greater range of motion at the elbow. Olecranon bursitis can be caused by trauma from a direct blow, chronic friction from prolonged leaning on the elbows, crystal deposition (gout), systemic diseases (rheumatoid arthritis, SLE, uremia), or infection [49–51]. It can be seen in sports such as football, wrestling, volleyball, and basketball [49,52]. Olecranon bursitis can present in one of three presentations: (1) acute, hemorrhagic bursitis due to direct trauma; (2) chronic, noninflamed bursal swelling associated with repetitive motions or rubbing of the elbow; and (3) an inflamed and possibly infected bursa [49].

Physical Examination

Patients present with a nontender, fluctuant bulge posterior to the olecranon process without decreased range of motion. Septic bursitis might present with fever, bursal warmth, tenderness in the center of the bursa, and peribursal cellulitis [50,51].

Diagnostic Studies

Radiographs are generally not necessary in acute bursitis but are helpful if fracture, dislocation, or ligament injury is suspected. Further imaging techniques, including bursography, ultrasonography, CT, or MRI, may be indicated for unresponsive cases or to exclude other causes. Aspiration of the fluid may be necessary if septic bursitis is suspected. This fluid should be sent for laboratory studies, including complete blood count, Gram stain, and culture. Gram-positive organisms, specifically *Staphylococcus aureus*, account for a majority of cases of septic bursitis [50].

Treatment

Most patients with olecranon bursitis can be treated non-operatively. Current expert opinion recommends ice, NSAIDs, and compressive dressing as initial treatment (grade of recommendation: D). Aspiration may be performed if the patient is symptomatic or if there is an urgency to return to play. Patients should be treated with antibiotics while awaiting culture results if septic bursitis is suspected. Intrabursal corticosteroid injections can be given for aseptic cases (grade of recommendation: D). Long-term treatment includes pads for the elbow, avoidance of inciting activity, ice, and NSAIDs. No studies exist regarding the efficacy of different treatment modalities.

Surgical intervention may be appropriate for individuals who fail needle aspiration or who have an inaccessible bursal site for repeated needle aspirations or in the presence of a foreign body or presence of necrotic tissue [50].

ROTATOR CUFF TENDINITIS

Clinical Presentation

Rotator cuff tendinitis is an injury that occurs in individuals participating in overhead activities, commonly involving swimmers, baseball pitchers, and heavy laborers. Patients present with posterolateral shoulder pain triggered with activities above the shoulder level. In addition, they may complain of pain with internal and external rotation that may affect their daily activities and note difficulty with sleeping on the affected side.

The shoulder pain associated with rotator cuff tendinitis typically occurs in patients between 50 and 70 years, is more common in women, and has an incidence from 10 to 20/1000 per year [53]. Rotator cuff tendinitis most commonly involves the supraspinatus tendon of athletes in their twenties and thirties or non-athletes who are older than 40 years [54,55].

The etiology of rotator cuff tendinitis is thought to be a combination of intrinsic and extrinsic factors. Intrinsic factors are injuries that originate within the tendon and include hypovascularity, age-related degeneration, and direct tendon overload. Extrinsic factors involve damage through compression against surrounding structures from bony impingement or soft-tissue pressure [53,54,56]. The differential diagnosis includes rotator cuff tear, subacromial bursitis, bicipital tendinitis, glenolabral tear, muscular strain, acromioclavicular sprain, and cervical radiculopathy [53,57].

Physical Examination

The physical examination begins with visual inspection to evaluate for symmetry, swelling, and atrophy, followed by testing active and passive range of motion. Most patients note a painful arc of motion between 60° and 120° of abduction.

Provocative tests focusing on specific structures assist with the diagnosis. Impingement signs, including the Neer and Hawkins tests, have been found to be positive in rotator cuff tendinitis. The Neer test involves passive forward flexion and medial rotation of the patient's arm, pushing the greater tuberosity against the anteroinferior border of the acromion. Reproduction of discomfort is considered a positive test. The Hawkins test involves forward flexion of the arm to 90° and medially rotating the shoulder, pushing the supraspinatus and biceps muscles against the inferior surface of the coracoacromial ligament and coracoid process [58].

Rotator cuff muscles can be easily tested during the physical examination. The supraspinatus muscle can be directly tested with the "empty can" or "Jobe" test. This involves placing the shoulder at 90° abduction, forward flexion of 30°, and medially rotating with the thumb pointing downward. Resistance against further flexion resulting in discomfort and demonstrating weakness is considered a positive test. Infraspinatus and teres minor can be tested with external rotation against resistance. The subscapularis muscle can be tested with the "lift-off" sign. The patient places the dorsum of the hand against the lumbar spine and is asked to lift the hand away from the back. Inability to complete this maneuver suggests subscapularis pathology. This test can be modified by placing resistance on the palm, with pain or weakness considered a positive test.

For additional diagnostic information, a subacromial injection of anesthetic may be used to differentiate between tendinitis and tear. A patient with tendinitis should be able to provide almost full resistance to strength testing after injection, whereas continued weakness is noted if a rotator cuff tear is present.

Diagnostic Studies

Plain radiographs are not needed for the initial evaluation of shoulder pain in the primary care setting unless trauma has occurred or the symptoms have been present for a prolonged period of time. The shoulder series should include an AP, internal and external rotation, scapular Y, and axillary lateral views. These images can reveal calcific deposits in the subacromial space or insertion of supraspinatus tendon, degenerative changes of the glenohumeral and acromioclavicular joints, narrowing of acromiohumeral space, and sclerosis and cyst-like changes at the greater tuberosity [53,55,59].

MRI is not routinely indicated in the primary care evaluation of shoulder pain and is often used before surgical consultation. Ultrasound has been used for diagnosis, providing a noninvasive and cost-effective tool. This diagnostic study is highly operator dependent. The tendon appears thickened, heterogenous, and abnormally hypoechoic [40,60].

Treatment

Initial treatment for rotator cuff tendinitis includes rest, icing, oral anti-inflammatory medication, and a rehabilitation program to strengthen rotator cuff muscles. Rehabilitation exercises initially emphasize restoring shoulder motion, followed by strengthening, proprioceptive training, and then returning to task or sport-specific activities [57]. A Cochrane review found weak evidence supporting (1) exercise for rotator cuff disease, with additional benefit from exercise plus mobilization, and (2) benefit of a supervised exercise regime (grade of Recommendation: C) [61].

A subacromial injection of corticosteroid may be considered for individuals with persistent symptoms. Little evidence exists to support or refute the efficacy of steroid injections (grade of recommendation: D) [62,63].

Surgical evaluation should be considered for individuals with symptoms that persist after completing a therapy program. Usually, nonsurgical therapy is recommended for at least 6 months. The surgeon may want to explore arthroscopically for other pathology, debride the tendon if necessary, or perform subacromial decompression.

Key Points

- Injuries commonly occur due to overuse, misuse, and underlying disease.
- Overuse injuries make up the most common subtype affecting athletes.
- The majority of injuries can be treated nonoperatively.

References

[1] Nirschl RP, Kreuscher BS. Assessment and treatment guidelines for elbow injuries. Physician Sports Med 1996;24.
[2] O'Connor FG, Howard TM, Fieseler CM, et al. Managing overuse injuries: a systematic approach. Physician Sports Med 1997;25.

[3] Wilder RP, Sethi S. Overuse injuries: tendinopathies, stress fractures, compartment syndrome, and shin splints. Clin Sports Med 2004;23:55–81.

[4] Meals R. De Quervain tenosynovitis. Available at: www.emedicine.com/orthoped/byname/de-quervain-tenosynovitis.htm. Accessed October 17, 2004.

[5] Kale S. Trigger finger Available at: www.emedicine.com/orthoped/topic570.htm. Accessed October 17, 2004.

[6] Patel MR, Bassini L. Trigger fingers and thumb: when to splint, inject, or operate. J Hand Surg [Am] 1992;17:110–3.

[7] Marks MR, Gunther SF. Efficacy of cortisone injection in treatment of trigger fingers and thumbs. J Hand Surg [Am] 1989;14:722–7.

[8] Fauno P, Anderson HJ, Simonson O. A long-term follow-up of the effect of repeated corticosteroid injections for stenosing tenosynovitis. J Hand Surg [Br] 1989;14:242–3.

[9] Jebson P, Kasdan M. Hand secrets. 2nd edition. Philadelphia: Hanley and Belfus; 2002, p. 71–3, 204.

[10] Richie CA, Briner W. Corticosteroid injection for treatment of de Quervain's tenosynovitis: a pooled quantitative literature evaluation. J Am Board Fam Pract 2003;16:102–6.

[11] Weiss AP, Akelman E, Tabatabai M. Treatment of de Quervain's disease. J Hand Surg [Am] 1994;19:595–8.

[12] Harvey F, Harvey P, Horsley M. De Quervain's disease: surgical or nonsurgical treatment. J Hand Surg [Am] 1990;15:83–7.

[13] Witt J, Pess G, Gelberman RH. Treatment of de Quervain tenosynovitis. J Bone Joint Surg Am 1991;73:219–22.

[14] Handoll HHG, Vaghela MV. Interventions for treating mallet finger injuries (Cochrane review). In: The Cochrane library, issue 3. Chichester, UK: John Wiley & Sons; 2004.

[15] Goodyear-Smith F, Arroll B. What can family physicians offer patients with carpal tunnel syndrome other than surgery? A systematic review of nonsurgical management. Ann Fam Med 2004;2:267–73.

[16] Jarvik JG, Yuen E, Haynor DR, et al. MR nerve imaging in a prospective cohort of patients with suspected carpal tunnel syndrome. Neurology 2002;58:1597–602.

[17] Steele M. Carpal tunnel syndrome. Available at: www.emedicine.com/emerg/topic83.htm. Accessed October 17, 2004.

[18] Viera A. Management of carpal tunnel syndrome. Am Fam Physician 2003;68:265–72.

[19] Ahn DS. Hand elevation: a new test for CTS. Ann Plast Surg 2001;46:120–4.

[20] O'Gradaigh D. A diagnostic algorithm for carpal tunnel syndrome based on Bayes's theorem. Rheumatology 2000;39:1040–1.

[21] Fuller DA. Carpal tunnel syndrome. Available at: www.emedicine.com/orthoped/topic455.htm. Accessed October 17, 2004.

[22] Jablecki CK, Andary MT, Floeter MK, et al. Practice parameter: electrodiagnostic studies in carpal tunnel syndrome. Report of the American Association of Electrodiagnostic Medicine, American Academy of Neurology, and the American Academy of Physical Medicine and Rehabilitation. Neurology 2002;58:1589–92.

[23] El Miedany YM, Aty SA, Ashour S. Ultrasonography versus nerve conduction study in patients with carpal tunnel syndrome: substantive or complimentary tests? Rheumatology 2004;43:887–95.

[24] Kele H, Verheggen R, Bittermann HJ, et al. The potential value of ultrasonography in the evaluation of the carpal tunnel syndrome. Neurology 2003;61:389–91.

[25] Jarvik JG, Yuen E, Kliot M. Diagnosis of carpal tunnel syndrome: electrodiagnostic and MR imaging evaluation. Neuroimaging Clin N Am 2004;14:93–102.

[26] Mesgarzadeh M, Schneck CD, Bonakdarpour A, et al. Carpal tunnel: MR imaging. Part II. Carpal tunnel syndrome. Radiology 1989;171:749–54.

[27] Radack DM, Schweitzer ME, Taras J. Carpal tunnel syndrome: are the MR findings a result of population selection bias? Am J Roentgenol 1997;169:1649–53.

[28] O'Connor D, Marshall S, Massy-Westropp N. Non-surgical treatment (other than steroid injection) for carpal tunnel syndrome (Cochrane review). In: The Cochrane library, issue 3. Chichester, UK: John Wiley & Sons; 2004.

[29] Gerritsen AA, de Krom MC, Struijs MA, et al. Conservative treatment options for carpal tunnel syndrome: a systematic review of randomized controlled trials. J Neurol 2002;249: 272–80.

[30] Marshall S, Tardif G, Ashworth N. Local corticosteroid injection for carpal tunnel syndrome (Cochrane review). In: The Cochrane library, issue 3. Chichester, UK: John Wiley & Sons; 2004.

[31] Wong SM, Hui AC, Tang A, et al. Local vs. systemic corticosteroids in the treatment of carpal tunnel syndrome. Neurology 2001;56:1565–7.

[32] Verdugo RJ, Salinas RS, Castillo J, et al. Surgical versus non-surgical treatment for carpal tunnel syndrome (Cochrane review). In: The Cochrane library, issue 3. Chichester, UK: John Wiley & Sons; 2004.

[33] Scholten RJPM, Gerritsen AAM, Uitdehaag BMJ, et al. Surgical treatment options for carpal tunnel syndrome (Cochrane review). In: The Cochrane library, issue 3. Chichester, UK: John Wiley & Sons; 2004.

[34] Nirschl RP, Ashman ES. Elbow tendinopathy: tennis elbow. Clin Sports Med 2003;22: 813–36.

[35] Peters T, Baker CL. Lateral epicondylitis. Clin Sports Med 2001;20:549–63.

[36] Ciccotti MG, Charlton WP. Epicondylitis in the athlete. Clin Sports Med 2001;20:77–93.

[37] Galloway M, DeMaio M, Mangine R. Rehabilitative techniques in the treatment of medial and lateral epicondylitis. Orthopaedics 1992;15:1089–96.

[38] Gruchow HW, Pelletier D. An epidemiologic study of tennis elbow: incidence, recurrence, and effectiveness of prevention strategies. Am J Sports Med 1979;7:234–8.

[39] Leach RE, Miller JK. Lateral and medial epicondylitis of the elbow. Clin Sports Med 1987;6:259.

[40] Jacobson J. Ultrasound in sports medicine. Radiol Clin N Am 2002;40:363–86.

[41] Assendelft W. Tennis elbow. Clin Evid Concise 2003;10:280–1.

[42] Smidt N, van der Windt DA, Assendelft WJ, et al. Corticosteroid injections, physiotherapy, or a wait and see policy for lateral epicondylitis: a randomized controlled trial. Lancet 2002;359:657–62.

[43] Brosseau L, Casimiro L, Milne S, et al. Deep transverse friction massage for treating tendinitis (Cochrane review). In: The Cochrane library, issue 3. Chichester, UK: John Wiley & Sons; 2004.

[44] Struijs PAA, Smidt N, Arola H, et al. Orthotic devices for the treatment of tennis elbow (Cochrane review). In: The Cochrane library, issue 3. Chichester, UK: John Wiley & Sons; 2004.

[45] Assendelft WJ, Hay EM, Adshead R, et al. Corticosteroid injections for lateral epicondylitis: a systematic overview. Br J Gen Pract 1996;46:209–16.

[46] Buchbinder R, Green S, White M, et al. Shock wave therapy for lateral elbow pain (Cochrane review). In: The Cochrane library, issue 3. Chichester, UK: John Wiley & Sons; 2004.

[47] Green S, Buchbinder R, Barnsley L, et al. Acupuncture for lateral elbow pain (Cochrane Review). In: The Cochrane Library Issue 4. Chichester, UK: John Wiley & Sons, Ltd.

[48] Buchbinder R, Green S, Bell S, et al. Surgery for lateral elbow pain (Cochrane review). In: The Cochrane library, issue 3. Chichester, UK: John Wiley & Sons; 2004.

[49] McFarland EG, Gill HS, Laporte D, et al. Miscellaneous conditions about the elbow in athletes. Clin Sports Med 2004;23:743–63.

[50] Valeriano-Marcet J, Carter JD, Vasey FB. Soft tissue disease. Rheum Dis Clin North Am 2003;29:77–88.

[51] Foye P. Olecranon Bursitis. Available at: www.emedicine.com/pmr/topic91.htm. Accessed October 17, 2004.

[52] Chumbley E. Evaluation of overuse elbow injuries. Am Fam Physician 2000;61:691–700.

[53] Mehta S, Gimbel J, Soslowsky LJ. Etiologic and pathogenetic factors for rotator cuff tendinopathy. Clin Sports Med 2003;22:791–812.

[54] Almekinders LC. Impingement syndrome. Clin Sports Med 2001;20:491–504.

[55] Browning D, Desai M. Rotator cuff injuries and treatment. Prim Care 2004;31:807–29.

[56] Blevins FT, Hayes WM, Warren RF. Rotator cuff injury in contact athletes. Am J Sports Med 1996;24:263–7.

[57] Bowen JE. Rotator cuff tendinitis. In: Frontera WR, editor. Essential of physical medicine and rehabilitation. 1st edition. Philadelphia: Hanly and Belfus; 2002. p. 83–9.

[58] Magee D. Shoulder. In: Magee DJ, editor. Orthopedic physical assessment. 4th edition. Philadelphia: WB Saunders; 2002. 263, 278–80.

[59] Talia AF, Cardone DA. Diagnostic and therapeutic injection of the shoulder region. Am Fam Physician 2003;67:1271–8.

[60] Morrey B, Regan W. Tendinopathies about the elbow. In: Delee J, Drez D, Miller MD, editors. DeLee and Drez's orthopaedic sports medicine. 2nd edition. Philadelphia: WB Saunders; 2003. p. 890–3.

[61] Green S. Physiotherapy interventions for shoulder pain (Cochrane review). In: The Cochrane library, issue 4. Chichester, UK: John Wiley & Sons; 2004.

[62] Buchbinder R. Corticosteroid injections for shoulder pain (Cochrane review). In: The Cochrane library, issue 4. Chichester, UK: John Wiley & Sons; 2004.

[63] Speed C. Shoulder pain. Clin Evid 2003;10:277–9.

Address reprint requests to

Rajwinder S. Deu, MD
Department of Family Medicine
Thomas Jefferson University
1015 Walnut Street, Suite 401
Philadelphia, PA 19107

e-mail: rajwinder.deu@mail.tju.edu

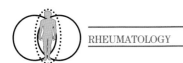
NEW TECHNOLOGY, NEW INJURIES IN THE HIP/GROIN

Jennifer Naticchia, MD, and Eshwar Kapur, MD

CURRENT CONCEPTS IN HIP AND GROIN INJURIES

Many musculoskeletal injuries are common and therefore familiar to the primary care physician. Various tendinopathies, ligament sprains, fractures, and acute exacerbations of osteoarthritis are seen frequently enough that repetition facilitates accurate diagnosis and treatment. Even more seemingly complicated diagnoses, such as SCL tear and Achilles tendon rupture, can be identified by providers who do not have a specific interest or added experience in sports medicine. Meanwhile, as sports-related physical activity has become more competitive and therefore arguably more intense and as more sophisticated imaging modalities have been developed, other conditions are being seen with significant frequency, some of which are more difficult to diagnose. With the progression of the field of sports medicine, further understanding of more recently identified medical conditions have allowed specialists to better diagnose patients, especially those who have failed conventional treatments in obscured clinical scenarios. Osteitis pubis (pubic symphysitis), microscopic or sportsman's hernia, and bone contusions are showing enough prominence and prevalence among hip and groin injuries that they should become better understood by family physicians, especially those taking care of athletes in any capacity. These are among the conditions considered in new paradigms of thought and are not immediately included in the differential diagnoses

From the Department of Family and Community Medicine, Christiana Care Health System, Wilmington, Delaware; and Primary Care Sports Medicine, Department of Family Medicine, Jefferson Medical College, Thomas Jefferson University, Philadelphia, Pennsylvania

The authors declare that they have no affiliation or financial interest in any organization that may have direct interest in the subject matter of this article.

and therefore often overlooked, thereby confounding treatment courses and complicating return to activity. This article discusses the importance of each of these conditions and introduces diagnostic and treatment protocols in the context of primary care. Although there is little evidence-based sports medicine and musculoskeletal injury literature, this article summarizes what is available. More evidence-based literature is needed.

SPORTS HERNIA

General

Groin pain is a significant complaint among athletes across a wide spectrum of sports, comprising up to 5% of all athletic injuries [1]. Muscle strains, particularly involving adductor musculature, are among the most likely causes of groin pain in athletes. The anatomy in the groin region is complex, and its central location mandates an expansive differential diagnosis that must include consideration of referred pain from the abdomen, spine, and reproductive organs. With chronic groin pain, a carefully focused history and clinical examination combined with judiciously ordered diagnostic testing often yields a working diagnosis and treatment plan. For unremitting symptoms, sports hernia (also known as microscopic or athlete's hernia) or athletic pubalgia should be considered in patients with chronic groin pain without clear cause. Typically, the diagnosis of sports hernia as a cause of chronic groin pain can be elusive because of its unfamiliarity among physicians and its paucity of physical findings. Because symptomatology in the groin can emanate from multiple coinciding processes [2], suspicion should be raised when a patient with a seemingly obvious diagnosis fails to improve with appropriate treatment. Therefore, a better understanding of the pathology, diagnosis, and treatment of athletic hernia is imperative for any physician caring for patients with musculoskeletal problems.

Definition and Pathophysiology

Direct and indirect inguinal hernias involve palpable defects located anteriorly toward the body surface, but the sports hernia is not visible or palpable on examination, occurring as an occult phenomenon. Although sports hernia represents a constellation of pathologic entities involving the inguinal canal [3,4], it has classically been defined as a nonpalpable defect in the integrity of the posterior inguinal wall [5,6] caused by weakness [5] or disruption. The posterior inguinal wall consists primarily of the transversalis fascia, along with the conjoint tendon, made up of the internal abdominal oblique and transversus abdominus aponeuroses. The absence of striated muscle at the posterior inguinal wall is thought to represent vulnerability in strength and therefore predispose the formation of a hernia [7]. It has been postulated that adductor muscle group contraction creates shearing forces that induce stress at this area of weakness [5].

There has been variability in the discussion of the musculature involved in the sports hernia. There have been several distinct descriptions of sports-related hernia acknowledging an array of possible locations, including the transversalis fascia or conjoint tendon [1,5], the internal oblique aponeurosis [8], and the external oblique aponeurosis [9]. Meanwhile, "hockey groin" has been described in professional hockey players, with herniation of the external oblique aponeurosis causing entrapment of the ilioinguinal nerve [10]. The common finding for all of these hernias is their occult nature. They are nonpalpable because of their posterior orientation or their microscopic size.

Differential Diagnosis

The differential diagnosis of groin pain can be divided into pathology within the groin and outside the groin. In the region of the groin, striated muscle strain, especially in the adductors, represents a common etiology of pain. Although muscle strains are usually acute, they can linger and become a chronic concern. Osteitis pubis and stress fractures in the pelvis can cause similar symptoms, and the more common indirect and direct hernias must be considered.

In the male reproductive system, infection, testicular mass, and torsion and other testicular injuries can cause pain radiating to the groin. Labral tears and avascular necrosis in the hip, lumbar radiculopathy in the spine, and osteoarthritis in the hip or spine are potential sources of groin pain. Other intra-abdominal pathology (eg, within the intestinal and renal systems from a variety of inflammatory, infectious, and other causes) can refer pain to the groin and should be considered when clinically compelling.

Clinical Examination

General Approach to Patients with Groin Pain

With the potential for significant losses in training and playing time and the possibility for excessive diagnostic testing, it is vital to effective disposition of the patient that the clinician effectively diagnose the athlete with chronic groin pain. Initially, it must be determined if the patient's pain is coming from the groin, the abdomen, the spine, the hips, or the reproductive organs. Also, although athletes likely have a musculoskeletal etiology of their symptoms, infectious, radicular, and various intra-abdominal causes should be considered. Multiple etiologies for groin pain should be considered that can complicate diagnosis [2].

History

Because the literature provides little guidance, patient history is the most important aspect of the evaluation of the athlete with groin pain (grade of recommendation: D). The clinician's understanding of the nature of the patient's symptoms is vital. Through a comprehensive interview, a clinician can significantly narrow the differential diagnosis by ruling out referred pain from nearby structures. Even within the region of the groin, elucidating an inciting event, relieving and exacerbating factors, and timing of pain can effectively direct a clinician toward an accurate diagnosis. Past medical and surgical history must be explored.

In the context of sports hernia, athletes typically describe unilateral pain during exercise that worsens over time. This pain is usually insidious in onset, although a significant number of athletes, especially soccer and hockey players, may be able to relate a sudden tearing sensation. Athletes involved in sports with repetitive twists, turns, and pivots at high speeds are at particular risk for sports hernia and describe pain worse with their activities. Runners, with minimal requirements for lateral movements or quick starts and stops, have been found with sports hernia as well. The duration of pain is typically months, and pain is usually resistant to conservative measures.

Physical Examination

The physical examination of the patient with groin pain is directed by the patient's history. Examination must include every area within the realm of the clinician's differential diagnosis, including the abdomen, reproductive organs, lower spine, pubic symphysis, and geographic musculature. The physical examination should improve the clinician's accuracy regardless of how certain the diagnosis initially seems.

A sports hernia is not palpable on abdominal or inguinal examination. Some clinicians have found that a dilated superficial inguinal ring may be palpated (grade of recommendation: D) [3]. There may be local tenderness superficially on lower abdomen palpation in the anatomic region. Pain reproducible with a sit-up could correlate with sports hernia (grade of recommendation: D) [3]. Any anterior involvement of a defect causing a sports-related hernia may present with findings or pain upon palpation in abdominal or inguinal examination. There is the potential for coexisting diagnoses, and physical examination findings may prove confusing when they suggest muscle strain or other more common diagnoses that do not improve with seemingly appropriate treatment.

Diagnostic Testing

Many athletes being evaluated for sports hernia have been evaluated and ruled out from most other more obvious or threatening conditions in the area. Testing could include x-ray, CT scan, and bone scan to evaluate surrounding bony pathology; MRI for soft tissue, intra-abdominal, or radicular causes; and MRI/MR arthrograms to rule out intra-articular hip pathology. Although these studies help to rule out alternate diagnoses, none is reliable in detecting sports hernias, although MRI may show related soft tissue pathologic findings.

There have been many studies assessing the utility of herniography for assisting in the diagnosis of sports hernia [11–15] and hernias in general [12]. The procedure, which involves an intraperitoneal injection of contrast dye followed by fluoroscopy or x-rays preferably with comparison to patient performing Valsalva maneuver, has been shown in a case series to find sports hernia but has limited sensitivity (grade of recommendation: C) [11]. Considering the substantial risk inherent in the procedure (complications including perforation occur in up to 5% [12–15]), one should exercise caution in recommending herniography and should take into account the experience and comfort of the radiologist with such a procedure. Dynamic ultrasonography has been found in certain case series to be useful in detecting various hernias (grade of recommendation: C) [7], including posterior wall defects [16], but such findings are highly operator dependent.

Treatment

Because of the paucity of findings on examination and the absence of an efficacious diagnostic test, there may be a tendency for physicians treating groin pain suspected to originate from a sports hernia to opt for an initial trial of conservative measures centered around rest from offending activities. Although this may be appropriate, especially if there is a coexisting diagnosis, consultation with a surgeon familiar with sportsman's hernia should be urged if suspected.

Surgery involves open or laparoscopic exploration for the exact defect and then some variation of repair, depending on the pathology. In case series in athletes with long-standing chronic groin pain suspected to emanate from sports hernia, return to play is variable but tends to be generally successful [4,10,17–19] (grade of recommendation: C) (Table 1). After surgery, patients should be enrolled in physical therapy for gradual stretching and strengthening of pelvic, groin, and hip musculature. Sudden movements should be avoided until sufficient healing has taken place.

TABLE 1.
Summary of Treatment Guidelines for Selected Hip/Groin Injuries

Condition	Proposed Treatment	Grade of Recommendation
Sports hernia	Surgical exploration and repair	C
Osteitis pubis	R.I.C.E + physical therapy	D
	Corticosteroid injection	C (athletes)
Bone contusions	Protection/relative rest	D

Recovery time varies according to the extent of surgery and should be directed by the operative physician.

OSTEITIS PUBIS

Osteitis pubis, or pubic symphysitis, is a painful inflammatory condition involving the pubic symphysis and surrounding structures. Its existence was described by Beer in 1924 [20], although it was first reported by urologists as a complication of suprapubic cystotomy in 1923 [21] and has been well documented as a complication of gynecologic and urologic surgery [21,22]. It was discussed in the context of athletes as early as 1932 and has more recently been frequently associated with athletes and active individuals [23–29]. Osteitis pubis should be recognized by primary care physicians as a possible cause for groin pain.

Differential Diagnosis

Box 1 highlights important musculoskeletal diagnoses that should be considered in the differential for groin pain. There are many systemic arthropathies and disease entities that should be considered in the differential diagnosis for groin pain; these diagnoses are not within the scope of this article, but many are described in this issue.

Pathophysiology

The pubic symphysis is a rigid nonsynovial amphiarthrodial joint consisting of layers of hyaline cartilage encasing a fibrocartilaginous disc [30]. It is hypothesized that shearing forces across the symphysis pubis cause inflammation in the pubic symphysis and the surrounding periosteum. Chronic inflammation from joint instability or other factors may lead to osteitis pubis [31]. Contributing factors to the general pathophysiology include repetitive adductor muscle contraction, sacroil-

---

Box 1. Differential Diagnosis for Osteitis Pubis/Groin Pain
- Adductor strain or tendonitis
- Abdominal muscle pull
- Adductor or abdominal muscle tear
- Inguinal hernia
- Sportsman hernia (microscopic hernia)
- Osteoarthritis of the hip
- Stress fracture (pubic, pelvic, or femoral)
- Iliac apophysitis
- Lumbar radiculopathy

iac joint instability, limitation in hip motion [32], and excessive pelvic motion [28]. Therefore, patients at risk for osteitis pubis include those who sustain repetitive extension of their lower abdomen and repetitive movements of the many muscles that attach to the pubic bone, especially the adductor muscles. Examples of athletic activity that may predispose an individual are ice hockey, soccer, running/sprinting, and American football, but any active person may present with this injury, and it must be considered in any patient with groin or hip pain [33,34].

Clinical Findings

Patients present to the primary care physician with pain in the groin or hip area. The pain can be unilateral or bilateral and has an insidious onset and progressively worsens. Other locations of the pain are medial thigh, testicular, scrotal, perineal and the suprapubic and anterior pubic areas. The pain is described as sharp and burning; less often, it is described as dull and achy. Exacerbating factors are activities that require the patient to extend his or her torso or simple weight-bearing exercises with additional pounding forces (eg, running). Activities potentially inducing pain include pivoting (especially one-legged pivoting), pushing off to change direction, twisting, doing sit-ups, doing leg raises, kicking, climbing stairs, and doing Valsalva maneuvers. It is difficult for the patient to lie in bed; an audible click may be heard by the patient with activities such as turning in bed or walking on uneven surface. This click may be explained by instability in the pubic symphysis. The authors advocate conventional treatment course consisting of rest, ice, heat, and anti-inflammatories and analgesics to relieve symptoms [33,34]. A detailed history allows the clinician to exclude systemic conditions considered in the differential diagnosis.

Physical examination helps to rule out many of the differential diagnoses. The most obvious and specific finding on physical examination is tenderness of the pubic bone upon palpation. More specifically, the patient can have tenderness upon palpation of the superior pubic rami (where the rectus abdominus muscles insert) or the inferior pubic rami (where the adductors attach). Hip range of motion can be restricted because of surrounding muscle spasm, especially of the adductors. Hip range of motion, active and passive, can elicit pain. Other provocative testing of the hip, including the lateral pelvic compression test and cross-leg test, can be positive. A positive Trendelenburg test indicates weak hip abductors. In severe cases, a patient can have a gait disturbance, specifically a wide-based (antalgic) gait disturbance with the hips and knees partially flexed [34].

Imaging

Standard plain AP and lateral radiographs of the pelvis rule out other potential causes and may assist in the diagnosis of osteitis pubis in symptomatic patients. The radiographic findings in osteitis pubis include varying amounts of subchondral irregularity with focal demineralization along with subchondral cysts or erosions [35]; however, these findings are not specific to osteitis pubis. Also, such findings on plain radiographs can lag behind clinical symptoms by as much as 4 weeks. Flamingo views reveal possible pubic joint hypermobility [35]. Sacroiliac joint films are recommended because this joint can be involved in the pathology [34]. Symphysography, with the injection of nonionic contrast into the symphysis pubis, can confirm osteitis pubis. The local anesthetic used to prepare the patient for contrast injection can invoke symptom reduction and therefore identify the pain source (grade of recommendation: D) [35].

MRI of the pelvis shows more detailed features of osteitis pubis, such as diffuse para-articular bone marrow edema or symphyseal disc extrusion [35]. A bone scan can also confirm the diagnosis. Such testing can be useful if the patient does not respond as expected to treatment but is typically ordered to rule out other causes of symptoms, including systemic illness or osteomyelitis.

Treatment and Prognosis

Osteitis pubis is generally thought of as a self-limiting condition. Because primary care physicians are not always aware of this diagnosis, some of the many conditions described previously are considered. This causes a delay in treatment and thus sets the patient back in his or her training, workouts, or activities of daily living. A multifactorial approach, incorporating the avoidance of inciting activities and the use of physical therapy to stretch and strengthen musculature surrounding the hip joints, leads to resolution in most cases (grade of recommendation: D). Ice and analgesics are thought to be effective adjunctive therapies and are generally recommended (grade of recommendation: D). Because of the question of inflammation versus joint degeneration/instability as possible causative factors, the use of nonsteroidal anti-inflammatories, oral corticosteroids, and corticosteroid injections is controversial. Intra-articular steroid injections have been used with variable results; several nonrandomized trials have suggested anecdotal-quality positive results in highly selective athletic patient populations (grade of recommendation: C) [28,35] (see Table 1). Future well-designed study protocols should provide further guidance on treatment efficacy.

Although there are limited data validating surgical stabilization, a recent study documented excellent results in a small group of athletes [31], and surgery could be considered in patients with persistent symptoms despite the exhaustive use of conservative measures (grade of recommendation: C).

BONE CONTUSIONS

Bone contusions are relatively common in musculoskeletal injury and are often associated with soft-tissue pathology. Bone contusion patterns can describe the mechanism of certain events, such as patellar dislocation and ACL sprain. Bone contusions are found in the absence of other pathology and can be responsible for symptoms in certain patients. It is unclear how bone contusions affect prognosis, treatment, and return to play. With the improved resolution of diagnostic studies such as MRI that have confirmed the frequent occurrence of bone contusions, the primary care provider should understand what a bone contusion is and its significance in the context of any associated injury. Animal studies suggest an association between bone contusion and eventual degenerative disease [36]. Although there are no human studies to confirm or challenge this finding, physicians should recognize that possible long-term implications should be acknowledged. Bone contusions occur in the hip and other areas vulnerable to contact, especially areas with less overlying cushioning soft tissue. Nevertheless, the information generated thus far in the literature originates from data collected from knee studies.

Pathophysiology

Bone contusions are caused by direct impact to bone. Disruption within the trabecular bone network (microfractures), with corresponding bone marrow edema and hemorrhage, are seen in histologic studies [37]. Bone marrow edema has been shown to correlate with pain due to increased intraosseous pressure as fluid accumulates [38]. Bone contusions and stress fractures can look similar, but history of trauma versus overuse, respectively, distinguishes one from the other [39]. There are varying types of bone contusions; the more severe lesions, in close proximity to subchondral bone, may cause eventual osteochondral pathology [40].

Clinical Findings

Patients with MRI findings consistent of bone contusions relate a history of a direct trauma onto the injured bone. They relate pain in the region of the trauma and have tenderness to palpation in this area on examination. There is a correlation in the knee between bone contusions and ligamentous injury [38,41–45], and studies demonstrate that bone contusions can occur alone as well [46]. Generally, careful clinical examination combining palpation, muscle strength, and ligament laxity testing as appropriate helps determine the existence of bony tenderness with or without associated soft-tissue damage.

Imaging

Although plain radiographs and CT helps rule out fracture, MRI is the mainstay in identifying bone contusions. T2 MRI images show a speckled appearance, and T1 images show decreased signal intensity [47], without evidence of fracture. Bone scintigraphy may show increased uptake to help confirm the diagnosis [39]. Radiographs taken 6 to 12 weeks postinjury may show focal degeneration [48].

Treatment and Prognosis

The natural history of bone bruises is largely unknown. Based on a return to normal appearance on MRI, bone contusions can resolve anywhere from less than 6 weeks to 2 to 4 months (level of evidence: 4) [44,49]. There are no studies to correlate pain with severity or existence of a bone contusion, and no studies have been designed to determine if any treatments could definitively shorten the natural course of injury, but a common-sense regimen of protection and relative rest would seem prudent (grade of recommendation: D) (see Table 1). Keeping that in mind with the mechanism for pain elicited from bone bruising, it is reasonable that there can be some confusion in determining the source of a patient's pain when there is associated soft tissue injury. This is especially true when evaluating a patient for possible surgery because of the lack of resolution of symptoms presumed from the sprained ligament. Therefore, it is important to consider the existence of a bone contusion in treatment decision-making.

Bone contusions generally have a benign course. With the possible association of bone contusions with osteochondral lesions and possible degenerative changes documented in animal studies, there is also a long-term prognostic concern. Physicians should be aware of the potential complications inherent in bone contusions to best advise patients.

Key Points

- Sports hernia is defined as any nonpalpable defect in the inguinal canal, commonly located posteriorly.
- Sports hernia is primarily a clinical diagnosis confirmed with surgical exploration.
- Surgical repair is the only definitive treatment for sports hernia.
- Osteitis pubis is an inflammatory process affecting the pubic symphysis and the surrounding periosteum.
- Osteitis pubis can be diagnosed by MRI or bone scan in conjunction with careful clinical examination.
- Appropriate conservative therapy for osteitis pubis can expedite resolution in this generally self-limited condition.
- Bone contusion is a potential source of symptoms in patients with otherwise normal clinical and diagnostic findings.
- MRI provides diagnostic evidence of bone contusions.
- Bone contusions are self-limiting and resolve with activity modification.

References

[1] Renstrom P, Peterson L. Groin injuries in athletes. Br J Sports Med 1980;14:30–6.
[2] Ekberg O, Persson NH, Abrahamsson PA, et al. Longstanding groin pain in athletes: a multidisciplinary approach. Sports Med 1988;6:56–61.
[3] Kemp S, Batt ME. The "sports hernia.". Phys Sportsmed 1998;26:36–44.
[4] Kumar A, Doran J, Batt ME, et al. Results of inguinal canal repair in athletes with sports hernia. J R Coll Surg Edinb 2002;47:561–5.
[5] Hackney RG. The sports hernia: a cause of chronic groin pain. Br J Sports Med 1993;27: 58–62.
[6] Joesting DR. Diagnosis and treatment of sportsman's hernia. Curr Sports Med Rep 2002;1:121–4.
[7] Fon LJ, Spence RAJ. Sportsman's hernia. Br J Surg 2000;87:545–52.
[8] Simonet WT, Saylor HL III, Sim L. Abdominal wall muscle tears in hockey players. Int J Sports Med 1995;16:126–8.
[9] Gilmore J. Groin pain in the soccer athlete: fact, fiction, and treatment. Clin J Sports Med 1998;17:787–93.
[10] Irshad K, Feldman LS, Lavoie C, et al. Operative management of "hockey groin syndrome": 12 years of experience in National Hockey League players. Surgery 2001;130: 759–66.
[11] Gwanmesia II, Walsh S, Bury R, et al. Unexplained groin pain: safety and reliability of herniography for the diagnosis of occult hernias. Postgrad Med J 2001;77:250–1.
[12] Calder F, Evans R, Neilson D, et al. Value of herniography in the management of occult hernia and groin pain in adults. Br J Surg 2000;87:824–5.
[13] Ducharme JC, Bertrand R, Chacar R. Is it possible to diagnose inguinal hernia by X-ray? A preliminary report on herniography. J Can Assoc Radiol 1967;18:448–51.
[14] Hall C, Hall PN, Wingate JP, et al. Evaluation of herniography in the diagnosis of an occult abdominal wall hernia in symptomatic adults. Br J Surg 1990;77:902–6.
[15] Brierly RD, Hale PC, Bishop NL. Is herniography an effective and safe investigation? J R Coll Surg Edinb 1999;44:374–7.
[16] Orchard JW, Read JW, Neophyton J, et al. Groin pain associated with ultrasound finding of inguinal canal posterior wall deficiency in Australian Rules footballers. Br J Sports Med 1998;32:134–9.
[17] Paajanen H, Syvahuoko I, Airo I. Totally extraperitoneal endoscopic (TEP) treatment of sportsman's hernia. Surg Laparosc Endosc Percutan Tech 2004;14:215–8.
[18] Kluin J, den Hoed PT, van Linschoten R, et al. Endoscopic evaluation and treatment of groin pain in the athlete. Am J Sports Med 2004;32:944–9.
[19] Genitsaris M, Goulimaris I, Sikas N. Laparoscopic repair of groin pain in athletes. Am J Sports Med 2004;32:1238–42.
[20] Beer E. Periostitis of the symphysis and descending rami of the pubis following suprapubic operations. Int J Med Surg 1924;37:224–5.
[21] Stenchever M. Comprehensive gynecology. 4th edition. St. Louis: Mosby; 2001.
[22] Lentz SS. Osteitis pubis: a review. Obstet Gynecol Surv 1995;50:310–5.
[23] Harris NH, Murray RO. Lesions of the symphysis in athletes. BMJ 1974;4:211–4.
[24] Koch R, Jackson DW. Pubic symphysitis in runners. Am J Sports Med 1981;9:62–3.
[25] Fricker PA, Taunton JE, Ammann W. Osteitis pubis in athletes: infection, inflammation or injury? Sports Med 1991;12:266–79.
[26] Batt ME, McShane JM, Dillingham MF. Osteitis pubis in collegiate football players. Med Sci Sports Exerc 1995;27:629–33.
[27] Harris NH, Murray RG. Lesions of the symphysis pubis in athletes. J Bone Joint Surg 1974;56B:563–4.
[28] Holt MA, Keene JS, Graf BK, et al. Treatment of osteitis pubis in athletes: results of corticosteroid injections. Am J Sports Med 1995;23:601–6.
[29] Koch RA, Jackson DW. Pubic symphysitis in runners: a report of two cases. Am J Sports Med 1981;9:62–3.
[30] Gamble JG, Simmons SC, Freedman M. The symphysis pubis: anatomic and pathologic considerations. Clin Orthop 1986;203:261–72.

[31] Williams PR, Thomas DP, Downes EM. Osteitis pubis and instability of the pubic symphysis: when nonoperative measures fail. Am J Sports Med 2000;28:350–5.

[32] Williams JG. Limitation of hip joint movement as a factor in traumatic osteitis pubis. Br J Sports Med 1978;12:129–33.

[33] Disabella VN. Osteitis pubis. eMedicine Clinical Knowledge Base, Institutional Edition. Available at http://www.emedicine.com. Accessed October 1, 2004.

[34] Vitanzo PC, McShane JM. Osteitis pubis solving a perplexing problem. Physician Sportsmed 2001;29:33–8.

[35] O'Connell MJ, Powell T, McCaffrey NM, et al. Symphyseal cleft injection in the diagnosis and treatment of osteitis pubis in athletes. Am J Roentgenol 2002;179:955–9.

[36] Donohue JM, Buss D, Oegema TR Jr, et al. The effects of indirect blunt trauma on adult canine articular cartilage. J Bone Joint Surg Am 1983;65:948–57.

[37] Rangger C, Kathrein A, Frey C, et al. Bone bruise of the knee: histology and cryosections in 5 cases. Acta Orthop Scand 1998;69:291–4.

[38] Felson D, Chaisson CE, Hill CL, et al. The association of bone marrow lesions with pain in knee osteoarthritis. Ann Intern Med 2001;134:541–9.

[39] Hofmann S. Painful bone marrow edema of the knee: differential diagnosis and therapeutic concepts. Orthop Clin North Am 2004;35:321–33.

[40] Vellet AD, Marks PH, Fowler PJ, et al. Occult post-traumatic osteochondral lesions off the knee: prevalence, classification, and short-term sequelae evaluated with MR imaging. Radiology 1991;178:271–6.

[41] Marks PH, Goldenberg JA, Vezina WC, et al. Subchondral bone infractions in acute ligamentous knee injuries demonstrated on bone scintigraphy and magnetic resonance imaging. J Nucl Med 1992;33:516–20.

[42] Stein LN, Fischer DA, Fritts HM, et al. Occult osseous lesions associated with anterior cruciate ligament tears. Clin Orthop 1995;313:187–93.

[43] Spindler KP, Schils JP, Bergfeld JA, et al. Prospective study of osseous, articular and meniscal lesions in anterior cruciate ligament tears by magnetic resonance imaging and arthroscopy. Am J Sports Med 1993;21:551–7.

[44] Graf BK, Cook DA, De Smet AA, et al. "Bone bruises" on magnetic resonance imaging evaluation of anterior cruciate ligament injuries. Am J Sports Med 1993;21:220–3.

[45] Mair SD, Schlegal TF, Gill TJ, et al. Incidence and location of bone bruises after acute posterior cruciate ligament injury. Am J Sports Med 2004;32:1681–7.

[46] Snearly WN, et al. Lateral-compartment bone contusions in adolescents with intact anterior cruciate ligaments. Radiology 1996;198:205–8.

[47] DeLee J. DeLee and Drez's orthopaedic sports medicine. 2nd edition. New York: Elsevier; 2003.

[48] Sanders TG, Medynski MA, Feller JF, et al. Bone contusion patterns of the knee at MR imaging: footprint of the mechanism of injury. Radiographics 2000;20:S135–51.

[49] Miller MD, Osborne JR, Gordon WT, et al. The natural history of bone bruises: a prospective study of magnetic resonance imaging-detected trabecular microfractures in patients with isolated medial collateral ligament injuries. Am J Sports Med 1998;26:15–9.

Address reprint requests to

Jennifer Naticchia, MD
Residency Director, Department of Family and Community Medicine
Christiana Care Health System
1401 Foulk Road, Suite 100
Wilmington, DE 19803

e-mail: JNaticchia@christianacare.org

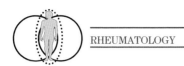
LOW BACK PAIN: A PRIMARY CARE APPROACH

Marc I. Harwood, MD, and Bradley J. Smith, MD

Low back pain (LBP) is a common ailment that affects a large portion of the population at one point or another. The lifetime prevalence of LBP pain has been reported to be 70% to 85%, and the annual prevalence of LBP has been estimated to be 15% to 45% [1]. LBP affects men and women equally, from their twenties into old age, and it is one of the leading causes for visits to a health care provider. Potential causes of LBP generate a vast differential diagnosis. Although the precise etiology may not be identified in up to 85% of patients, the majority of cases are thought to be due to muscular or ligamentous injuries that are usually self-limited [2]. The history and physical examination are important tools used to determine whether the etiology is among the benign causes of LBP or if there is a potentially more serious cause of LBP present [2,3].

LBP is common, but many individuals do not seek care for the condition. Patients who seek help present to a broad spectrum of providers, including primary care physicians, orthopedists, neurologists, acupuncturists, chiropractors, masseurs, and holistic healers. Carey et al [4] conducted a telephone survey of a random sample of households in North Carolina ($n = 3505$) and reported that approximately 7.6% of adult respondents had acute back pain (<3 months) that was functionally limiting over the past year. Of those who had pain, only 39% sought medical care from allopathic physicians, chiropractors, or other health care providers. Those who were more likely to seek medical care had more severe pain, more prolonged pain, or radicular symptoms (sciatica). Gender, age, income, health care status, and rural versus urban residency did not correlate with the decision to seek care [4].

From the Department of Family Medicine, Jefferson Medical College, Thomas Jefferson University, Philadelphia, Pennsylvania (MIH, BBJS); and the Sports Medicine Fellowship Program, Jefferson Medical College, Thomas Jefferson University, Philadelphia, Pennsylvania (MIH)

Patient history and physical examination are the most valuable tools used to risk-stratify patients. The goal on the initial evaluation of a patient is twofold. First, the physician must try to distinguish common mechanical back pain from a more serious problem, such as malignancy, infection, trauma, or substantial neurologic compromise (cauda equina syndrome or spinal cord compression). Although it is often difficult to find an exact cause of nonspecific back pain, more serious causes can be diagnosed with greater certainty through an appropriate history and physical examination. Additionally, although symptoms concerning for these more serious conditions can be readily identified, the prevalence of such causes is so low that, despite suggestive histories, most work-ups to confirm the suspicion demonstrate benign, nonspecific mechanical causes [2].

The second goal of the initial evaluation is to begin treatment in a manner designed to lessen the probability that a patient with acute LBP will progress to chronic back pain (defined as pain that lasts longer than 12 weeks), which is a different entity. Patients who have chronic back pain incur much higher costs on the health care system and on society, and it is of paramount importance to prevent this progression [5].

NATURAL HISTORY

The vast majority of cases of LBP recover spontaneously and without medical attention. The American Academy of Orthopaedic Surgeons reports that 90% of back pain patients seen in general practice are pain free within 3 months, and over 90% of those patients recover spontaneously within 4 weeks [6,7].

The first priority in treatment is to determine if the patient may safely start conservative therapy or if a diagnostic work-up is required to rule out systemic causes. The history and physical examination guide the physician to decide which patients need studies to evaluate and rule out more serious conditions. Most patients in the primary care setting do well after the initiation of therapy and undergo subsequent tests if progressive neurologic deficits are present or if there is failure to improve after 6 weeks. A suggested overall treatment strategy is provided in Fig. 1.

It is desirable to prevent the transition from acute or subacute LBP into chronic back pain, a condition that is responsible for the majority of health care expenditures related to LBP [8]. The pathophysiology of chronic LBP poorly understood. Many of these patients will never be completely pain free, so the treatment goal is to find a way to maximize functional ability.

DIAGNOSTIC APPROACH

The major diagnostic task facing the physician is to differentiate the patient with back pain that will resolve from patients with an underlying

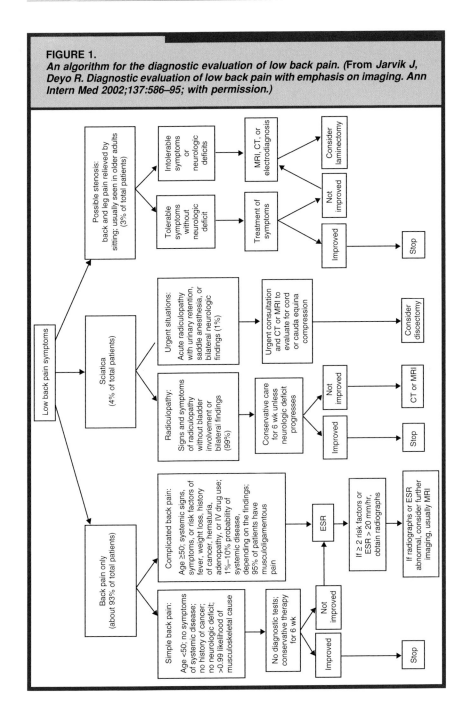

FIGURE 1.
An algorithm for the diagnostic evaluation of low back pain. (From Jarvik J, Deyo R. Diagnostic evaluation of low back pain with emphasis on imaging. Ann Intern Med 2002;137:586–95; with permission.)

serious disease or neurologic impairment. LBP can be broken down into three categories: (1) mechanical LBP, including lumbar strain/sprain, degeneration (osteoarthritis), disc herniation, spinal stenosis, and fracture (traumatic or compression); (2) nonmechanical conditions, including malignancy, infection, and inflammatory conditions; and (3) visceral disease (pain referred from other organs).

When first evaluating a patient with LBP, it is important to look for "red flags" that may indicate a more serious problem. Signs of neurologic compromise, including saddle anesthesia or bowel or bladder dysfunction (particularly urinary retention), may be indicative of spinal cord compression or cauda equina syndrome. The discovery of significant neurologic dysfunction necessitates emergent evaluation by CT or MRI and surgical consultation.

Infection may be present if there is fever or localized tenderness and warmth. Most infections are seeded by blood-borne pathogens from sites such as the urinary tract or the skin or are introduced by the injection of illicit drugs. Infectious causes of back pain are uncommon, accounting for approximately 0.01% of cases of LBP [9].

Another serious possibility is primary or metastatic malignancy, which is the cause of 0.7% of back pain [9]. Cancer is the most common systemic disease to cause back pain [3]. Risk factors include age > 50 years, unremitting pain, night pain, unexplained weight loss, or a personal history of previous cancer. If none of these is present, Deyo et al [9] report a combined sensitivity of 1.00 and specificity of 0.6 for the absence of cancer. Other historical factors that may help look for systemic clues are listed in Table 1. Patients with reason for concern should be evaluated by plain x-rays and screening labs to see if treatment must be altered.

Certain inflammatory processes can cause LBP, such as the spondyloarthropathies. These conditions (eg, ankylosing spondylitis) are more common in young men. They comprise a relatively small portion of LBP cases (0.3%). These conditions can present in a similar fashion to mechanical back pain [10]. However, inflammatory type pain classically presents differently from the pain from musculoskeletal injury (Box 1). Patients without the listed complaints or other symptoms of spondyloarthropathies (eg, uveitis, arthralgias, constitutional symptoms, etc.), are more likely to have mechanical back pain, especially if there is an identifiable causative event (pain suffered after lifting/working). Although there are characteristics suggestive of inflammatory back pain, they are poorly sensitive and specific to inflammatory back pain and are frequently found in patients with mechanical LBP.

It is well established that back pain and recovery are influenced by more than just anatomic problems. Patients injured at work tend to be disabled longer, although exact numbers have not been consistent between studies [11,12]. Individuals with workers' compensation claims or legal action also tend to take longer to return to work and use more medical resources (hazard ratio for attendance to work 0.53, 95% confidence interval [CI] 0.30–0.94) [13].

TABLE 1.
Diagnostic Accuracy of Historical Elements

Disease State	Historical clue	Sensitivity	Specificity
Cancer	Age ≥50 yr	0.77	0.71
	History of previous cancer	0.31	0.98
	Unexplained weight loss	0.15	0.94
	Failure to improve after 1 mo	0.31	0.90
	No relief with bed rest	> 0.90	0.46
Infection	Fever	0.27–0.83	0.98
	Spine tenderness	0.86	0.60
Compression fracture	Age ≥50 or 70 yr	0.84, 0.22	0.61, 0.96
	Trauma history	0.30	0.85
	Long-term corticosteroid use	0.06	0.995
Disk herniation	Sciatica/radicular symptoms	0.95	0.88
Spinal stenosis	Neurogenic claudication	0.60	N/A
	Age ≥50 yr	0.90	0.70

Adapted from Deyo RA, Rainville J, Kent DL. What can the history and physical examination tell us about low back pain? JAMA 1992;268:760–5; with permission.

HISTORY

The best initial diagnostic approach is to stratify the presenting complaint into certain categories while looking out for red flags. Most patients do not require diagnostic testing because the history and physical provide most of the requisite information [2]. The most important part of the patient's history is to determination if there are symptoms of urgent neurologic compromise (eg, bladder retention, saddle anesthesia), which would suggest cauda equina syndrome or cord compression. Patients with worrisome neurologic examinations must be imaged and evaluated by a surgeon quickly to prevent permanent damage.

Box 1. Patient Characteristics Suggestive of Spondyloarthropathy

- Onset of pain/discomfort before age 40
- Onset is insidious (slow, gradual onset)
- Duration of pain › 3 months
- Presence of morning stiffness
- Pain improves with exercise, movement

Data from Van der Linden S, van der Heijde D. Ankylosing spondylitis: clinical features. Rheum Dis Clin North Am 1998;24:663–76; with permission.

Once neurologic compromise is excluded, it is important to determine the location of the pain generator. Historical clues of aggravating factors can help. Pain that worsens with extension classically arises from the posterior aspects of the spine, such as spinal stenosis, degenerative disc disease, and facet arthropathy. This is in contrast with pain aggravated by forward flexion, which is classically related to anterior problems, such as ligamentous injury or disc herniation.

Many different problems produce musculoligamentous pain, and the character of the pain can help identify the pain generator [14]. Pain with a more gradual onset that worsens after resting or sitting may be myofascial LBP. This can be aggravated by cold and can be relieved with warmth and motion. Sharp, shooting pain that is aggravated by coughing, sneezing, and straining is more typical of pain from an irritated nerve root. Lying down classically relieves this neuropathic pain. Nocturnal pain or constant unremitting pain may represent malignancy or infection. Pain that radiates in a small area surrounding the injury with associated localized tenderness can be indicative of fractures of the thoracic or lumbar spine. Risk factors for fracture include trauma, strenuous lifting, prolonged corticosteroid use, or preexisting osteoporosis.

The majority of patients with LBP have discomfort confined to the low back, but some patients have radicular symptoms or pain that radiates into the lower extremity. Radicular pain can be attributed to any pathologic process within the spine that causes irritation of nerve roots. Although not all radicular pain is caused by disc herniation, radicular pain is sensitive for the presence of herniation (sensitivity 0.95, specificity 0.88), and its absence makes a clinically significant lumbar herniation and resultant nerve root irritation unlikely [9]. Pain that radiates into the buttocks and proximal thigh is not necessarily caused by nerve compression. Pain radiating down below the knee or into the foot, perhaps with associated paresthesias in a dermatomal distribution (radicular pain), is highly suggestive of nerve root compression [9].

Patients with spinal stenosis may experience neurogenic claudication, a syndrome in which pain radiates down the legs, particularly when walking, and is often relieved by rest. Spinal stenosis is a different entity from typical musculoligamentous LBP or pain from discogenic pain. In this condition, the stenosis, or narrowing of the spinal canal, is usually caused by hypertrophic degenerative changes in the spinal architecture. Commonly affected sites are the vertebral facets and the ligamentum flavum. The stenotic area can be central or in the lateral recesses of the canal [12]. Classically, this can be distinguished from vascular claudication because the pain of neurogenic claudication starts even while the patient stands still. The pain is worsened by extension of the spine, which occurs with standing or walking, and improves with flexion, such as sitting or leaning forward. Extension unloads the vertebral bodies and places more of a load on the facets, thus narrowing the neuroforaminal canals slightly. This is in contrast to discogenic pain, which is typically worsened by spinal flexion, which puts more weight over the anterior vertebral body and forces the disc posteriorly toward the canal.

Certain historical clues can raise clinical suspicion of spondylolysis and spondylolisthesis. Pain with extension of the spine in a young athlete should prompt the clinician to include spondylolysis in the differential diagnosis. This condition is caused by a defect in the pars interarticularis. The problem may be congenital or may be caused by a stress fracture. Adolescent athletes of sports that require hyperextension of the spine, such as gymnasts and football linemen, are the typical patients who experience this problem. Early recognition of spondylolysis and initiation of proper therapy can decrease the associated morbidity and speed return to activity [15].

If a stress fracture progresses, it can cause a complete fracture across the pars interarticularis and consequently destabilize the spine, allowing the superior vertebrae to move forward relative to the inferior vertebral body. The result is spondylolisthesis, or forward slippage of one vertebra relative to its adjacent vertebra. Spondylolisthesis can occur secondary to spondylolysis, but it may result from extensive degenerative disc disease, particularly in elderly individuals. These translational movements may cause narrowing of the neuroforamina, which leads to spinal stenosis [12]. For patients with a suggestive history, it is important to assess range of motion and tolerance of spinal flexion and extension.

PHYSICAL EXAMINATION

A standard approach to the physical examination can help the examiner find the most likely problem. The examination starts upon first seeing the patient. The clinician should take note of the patient's gait, posture, movement, and comfort level. Signs of neuromuscular damage can sometimes be seen, such as muscle atrophy or fasciculations. In addition to a neuromuscular evaluation, the examination should include assessment of the abdomen, peripheral pulses, hips, and inguinal areas. A rectal examination should be done if cauda equina is suspected because it may be evident by decreased anal tone.

The physician should inspect the spine before performing a neurologic examination. Abnormalities in curvature or development may be apparent. Cutaneous signs of deeper processes can often be seen, such as bruising, redness, swelling, or spinal variations. It is important to test the patient's range of motion at the waist, especially with forward flexion and backward extension. Movements that trigger the pain should be identified and tested. Palpation should be done over the spinous processes to try to elicit bony tenderness. Palpation directly over the vertebrae provides a force directed anteriorly, which may aggravate discogenic pain, spondylolisthesis, or injury to the longitudinal ligaments.

The straight leg raise test is an important diagnostic maneuver. The patient sits on a table with knees bent and leans forward slightly, flexing the spine and with the shoulders forward. This is our preferred method to perform a straight leg raise test (Fig. 2). The examiner grabs a foot and

FIGURE 2.
The seated straight-leg raise. The patient is asked to sit upright with the knees bent. (A) The spine and shoulders are flexed forward. (B) The examiner fully extends the leg at the knee. A positive test is reproduction of symptoms into the extended lower extremity (solid arrow). Classically, this maneuver causes a patient with nerve root irritation to adopt the tripod position (C), in which the back is extended to relieve the tension on the tethered, irritated nerve root.

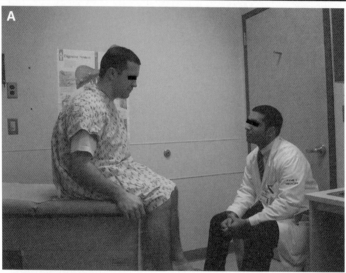

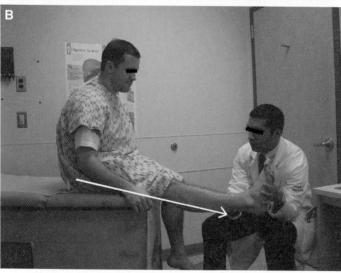

FIGURE 2 *(continued)*

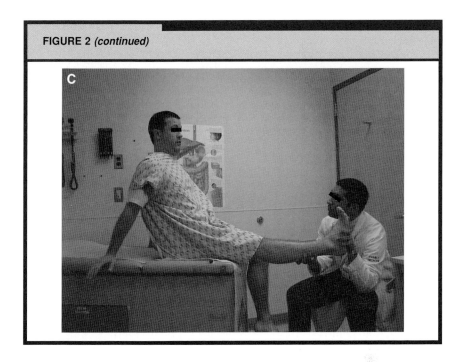

extends the leg upward (Fig. 2B). This maneuver—the straight leg raise test (SLR)—is designed to apply traction along the nerve root, which exacerbates pain if that nerve root is acutely inflamed. Traction can be increased by dorsiflexion at the ankle. Performing the test while the patient is seated gives fewer false-positives than the Lasegue's sign (raising the entire leg up while the patient lies supine), a test that results in more strain on the hamstrings. A positive test elicits pain in the leg, back, or buttocks at 60° or less of leg elevation. The sensitivity and specificity of the SLR are 0.80 and 0.40, respectively, for a clinically significant disc herniation [14]. In addition to supporting the diagnosis, a positive SLR can suggest where the lesion is located. A study by Xin et al [16] demonstrated that the distribution of pain occurring during the SLR allowed an accurate prediction of the anatomic location of the lesion 88.5% of the time.

The crossed SLR test is a variant of the SLR. In this maneuver, the radicular symptoms are reproduced in the symptomatic leg while the asymptomatic leg is raised. A positive SLR usually indicates a disc herniation medial to the nerve root, which may be accompanied by an extruded disc fragment. The crossed SLR test is less sensitive at detecting a clinically significant disc herniation than the regular test (0.25 versus 0.80 for the traditional SLR) but is more specific (0.90 versus 0.40 for the SLR) [14].

When assessing muscle strength, it is important to remember that the musculature in the lower extremity is supplied by the lumbar plexus,

TABLE 2.
Strength and Motor Testing to Evaluate Different Nerve Roots

Nerve Root	Reflex	Muscle	Test
L4	Knee jerk	Quadriceps	Leg extension weakness
L5	Hamstrings	Extensor Hallicus Longus	Weakness of great toe extension
		Tibialis anterior	Weakness of ankle dorsiflexion (possible foot drop)
S1	Ankle jerk	Gluteus maximus	Affected gait, pelvic tilt, weakness of hip external rotatorr
		Flexor digitorum	Weakness of toe flexors
		Gastrocnemius	Weakness of plantar flexion, weakness of heel-raise

which is comprised of nerves from more than one nerve root (Table 2). Consequently, a lesion at an isolated nerve root would cause weakness but not complete paralysis or atrophy; this would imply a lesion at multiple levels or damage to a peripheral nerve.

Radicular pain traveling down the leg typically follows an anatomic distribution depending on the nerve involved. Lumbar disc herniations occur 95% of the time at the L4-L5 or L5-S1 interspace, thereby affecting predominately the L5 and S1 nerve roots, respectively [17]. Radiculopathy involving the S1 nerve classically presents as leg pain worse than back pain, traveling from the buttock down the posterior thigh, along the posterolateral calf and heel into the lateral foot and fibular two toes [18]. Numbness or decreased sensation in this distribution may be present. The muscles supplied by the S1 nerve root follow a similar path. Weakness may be noted in the toe flexors, ankle dorsiflexors, toe abductors, and foot everters. The ankle jerk reflex may be decreased [14].

Nerve root involvement at L5 typically presents with more back than leg pain [14]. The pain and paresthesias classically travel down the posterolateral thigh, down the lateral calf, and into the dorsomedial foot and the tibial two toes. Weakened muscles from this injury can be found by testing the extensor hallices longus, the tibialis anterior and peronia muscles, and by impairing great toe extension and causing a foot drop. Reflex testing for L5, the hamstring jerk, is unreliable for the diagnosis of an L5 nerve root lesion because of innervation from more than one nerve root level. This is in contrast to the ankle jerk (S1) and the knee jerk (L4), which are predominantly supplied by the respective nerve roots [14].

Occasionally, the L4 nerve root is affected, causing LBP that radiates down the anteromedial thigh and knee. Sensation can be decreased in this area, and the knee jerk may be diminished or absent. Knee extension may be weaker than the contralateral side, but there is contribution from L3 to the quadriceps preserving some strength to this muscle.

It is important to compare one leg to the other to see if there are subtle differences. Proper use of torque and leverage can help the examiner determine if there is weakness in a muscle that is still relatively strong via secondary innervation. Muscle strength should be tested by placing the muscle in a mechanical disadvantage, such as extremes of flexion or extension.

LABORATORY EVALUATION

Laboratory studies are not needed in most patients. Laboratory studies can help eliminate potentially serious causes of pain from systemic disease in selected patients. Typical studies may include a complete blood count and erythrocyte sedimentation rate (ESR) if infection is suspected by the presence of constitutional symptoms or unremitting night pain. The ESR is elevated in approximately 80% to 90% of patients with osteomyelitis but is not a highly sensitive or specific marker if used as a screen for infection [19]. An elevated ESR in a patient with other supporting signs or symptoms should prompt further work-up. The ESR can also be followed as a marker for treatment. A prostate-specific antigen test may be useful in a patient with a history of prostate cancer in whom vertebral metastasis is suspected. A serum and urine protein electrophoresis may be considered if multiple myeloma is suspected [20]. The above laboratory tests are helpful if malignancy or infection is a potential causative agent. Otherwise, blood tests do not significantly change management of patients with LBP.

For most patients with LBP, a thorough history and physical examination is all that is needed to establish a likely diagnosis and initiate therapy. Waiting 4 weeks before ordering lab tests allows time for the large portion of normal LBP episodes to resolve spontaneously, therefore precluding the need for further work-up. After this time, it may be important to verify if there are other factors involved or if the treatment needs to be reassessed.

DIAGNOSTIC IMAGING

Most patients do not need radiographic imaging upon initial presentation. Imaging is helpful if there are suspicions of more serious underlying conditions or nerve compression that may need to be addressed surgically. For primary care physicians, the imaging modalities used most commonly are x-ray, MRI, and nuclear medicine bone scans. On occasion, subspecialists may obtain more advanced imaging with CT myelography, discography, and PET scans, but these are not usually needed in the majority of LBP work-ups; they are usually used when planning for surgery.

x-Rays are helpful to evaluate for fracture, osseous lesions, sacroiliitis, infection, and overall bony architecture. x-Rays should be included in the initial work-up if "red flags" are present or if the etiology of the LBP is believed to be nonmechanical. Simple anteroposterior and lateral views are more than sufficient in an initial evaluation of most

patients, forgoing the higher radiation exposure needed for oblique films
[3]. If a patient's complaints and history are suggestive of spondylolysis
(pain in active persons engaging in frequent extension), oblique views can
help assess this condition. If there is concern for instability in patients with
possible spondylolysis or spondylolisthesis or in patients with prior spinal
surgery, flexion and extension films should be obtained to look for forward
slippage of one vertebra over another [14].

Although CT scanning is often foregone in favor of MRI, CT scanning
does have its benefits. CT myelography is useful if surgical treatment is
being considered but should not generally be used as a diagnostic test in
the primary care setting. Due to the speed in which it can be obtained and
the detail in which it visualizes bone, CT is a preferred test in patients with
trauma to evaluate for fractures. CT is often considered if a patient has had
prior surgery of the lumbar spine and the resultant anatomy needs to be
defined [14].

MRI is a frequently used imaging modality in patients with back pain.
MRI requires no associated radiation and provides excellent image quality
of soft tissue structures compared with CT scans (Fig. 3). The pitfall of MRI
lies in its ability to define the anatomy, which invariably shows a deviation
from the "normal" musculoskeletal anatomy (eg, disc bulging, herniation,
or osteoarthritic changes). Caution should be used when interpreting the

FIGURE 3.
*(A) A sagittal T2 FSE MRI demonstrates a large L5–S1 disc herniation (solid
arrow). Note the absence of bright signal intensity at the L5–S1 interspace
(dashed arrow) in contrast to the interspaces at other levels, which denotes
marked disc desiccation. (B) An axial T2 FSE MRI demonstrates that the disc
herniation is asymmetric to the left. (Courtesy of D. Deely, MD, Philadelphia,
PA.)*

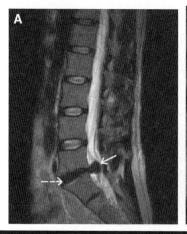
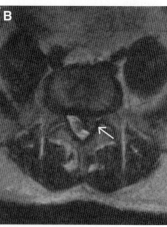

films because the identified problem may not be the source of pain. A study of lumbar spine MRI in asymptomatic individuals ($n = 98$) showed that 64% of patients without back pain had an intervertebral disc abnormality (disc bulge, protrusion, or herniation) [21]. Furthermore, 38% of the patients in the study had abnormalities at more than one level [21]. The LAIDBack study [22] prospectively followed a cohort of randomly selected Veterans Affairs outpatients ($n = 148$) to try to determine the prevalence of abnormal lumbar MRI findings in patients without LBP or radicular symptoms at the time of imaging. Of the 148 patients, 46% never experienced LBP before the study. A breakdown of abnormal MRI findings was as follows: 83% had moderate to severe desiccation of one or more discs, 64% had bulging discs, 32% had at least one protrusion, and 6% had one or more herniations [22]. The authors of that study concluded that many MRI findings have a high prevalence in patients without LBP, and, therefore, these findings are of limited diagnostic utility. A 7-year follow-up study of the same asymptomatic patients as used in 1990 [23] showed that anatomic problems seen on MRI in an asymptomatic patient do not imply that the patient will suffer from back pain in the future. Patients with no prior abnormalities were as likely to report having back pain as those with abnormalities on the original MRI scans. Additionally, several subjects that had abnormalities in 1990 and 1997 did not report ever having LBP before the original scans or at any point during the 7-year follow-up study.

MRI should be considered if there is any presence of bowel/bladder incontinence, sexual function deficits, or a history of lumbar spinal stenosis in the face of neurologic deficits. These patients may have cord compression or cauda equina syndrome and should be evaluated to see if surgical intervention is warranted. Most authors agree that radicular pain alone is not an indication for MRI scanning [3,12,14,21,23]. In patients with severe pain refractory to nonsurgical treatment or in patients with progressive neurologic deficits, further imaging should be considered.

Bone scans are nuclear studies that can be useful if cancer, osteomyelitis, or stress fractures are suspected. These studies are sometimes obtained if oblique x-rays raise the possibility of spondylolysis to ascertain if a stress fracture is present [15]. Bone scans are also useful when investigating for metastatic lesions in patients with a prior history of cancer.

NONSURGICAL THERAPY

Most patients presenting with LBP, including those with radicular symptoms, benefit from an initial trial of nonsurgical treatment. A summary of these treatments and recommendations is included in Table 3. The initial treatment plan includes changes in activity and pharmacologic therapies. Bed rest has been frequently prescribed, but current evidence does not support its use to treat LBP. Hagen et al [24] evaluated nine studies with a total of 1435 patients and reported no statistically significant difference in pain intensity in the short term (≤ 3 weeks) or the

TABLE 3.
Summary of the Nonsurgical Treatment Options for Low Back Pain

Treatment Modality	Recommendation	Grade of Recommendation	Comment
Bed rest	To be avoided	A	Bed rest should be avoided; patients should be instructed to remain as active as possible within the limits of their pain.
Lifestyle modification: weight loss, tobacco cessation, exercise program	Recommended	C	Limited evidence as these nonmedical therapies do not lend themselves to easy comparison and analysis via RCT.
Physical therapy	Recommended	D	Limited evidence to document efficacy, but most clinicians agree that PT should be routinely recommended.
NSAIDs	Recommended	A	Drugs of choice for management of acute LBP
Acetaminophen	Not routinely recommended	B	Inconsistent evidence suggests that NSAIDs may be superior to acetaminophen.
COX-2 inhibitors	Not recommended	B	No more efficacious than traditional NSAIDs. Have been touted for their beneficial GI side-effect profile; however, new data regarding prothrombotic risk is concerning.
Muscle relaxants	May be helpful for bothersome night symptoms	B	Can be helpful for short courses, but the benefit arises with significant side effects, particularly sedation.

Treatment	Recommendation	Grade	Comments
Narcotic analgesics	Recommended only for severe LBP	C	Studies comparing narcotics to NSAIDs and acetaminophen are of low quality. Narcotic analgesics may be helpful for severe cases of LBP with marked functional limitations.
Tramadol	Recommended for moderate-to-severe pain	A	Tramadol can be used as an adjunct to NSAIDs.
Epidural steroid injections	Recommended in carefully selected patients	D	Limited evidence for utility, but low methodologic quality of studies
Spinal manipulation	Not routinely recommended	C	No documented benefit, but a generally safe modality
Chiropractic manipulation	Not routinely recommended	D	Not more effective than other treatment modalities, but patient satisfaction is high with chiropractic treatment
TENS	Not routinely recommended	B	Limited evidence to support its use, but a safe modality
Prolotherapy	Not recommended	D	Evidence is lacking, and there are limited long-term data to document safety.
Acupuncture/massage	Not routinely recommended	B	No high-quality evidence available to support its use, but a generally safe modality.
Back School	Reserved for patients with chronic LBP with marked functional impairment	B	Cost-effectiveness data unavailable
Heat or cryotherapy	Recommended	C	No high-quality evidence to support its use. Safe, minimally invasive modality

Abbreviations: LBP, low back pain; NSAID, nonsteroidal anti-inflammatory drug; PT, physical therapy; RCT, randomized control trial.

intermediate term (3–12 weeks) for patients treated with bed rest as compared with maintaining activity (evidence level: 2; meta-analysis). The review demonstrated a short-term (<3 week) decrease in functional status for the bed rest group compared with the usual activity group as measured by a standardized disability questionnaire (mean decrease in functional status score 3.20, 95% CI 0.64–5.75, $P < 0.01$) [24]. Bed rest is not without its own risks, including deconditioning and venous thromboembolic events [25]. Therefore, bed rest does not relieve pain better when compared with maintaining activity, and it may lead to a decrease in function (grade of recommendation: A).

Hilde et al [26] report in a systematic review that providing medical advice to stay active as the lone treatment for LBP with radicular symptoms was an effective treatment for even without any other intervention (level of evidence: 1; systematic review). The treatment group advised to stay active had a small but statistically significant difference in functional status (as measured on a numeric scale 0–100, weighted mean difference [WMD] 6.0, 95% CI 1.5–10.5) and a shorter length of sick leave (WMD 3.4 days, 95% CI 1.6–5.2) as compared with the group prescribed bed rest [26]. The authors report that there is no evidence from available studies to suggest that staying active is harmful for LBP or radiculopathy. Patients should be encouraged to stay as active as they can tolerate, and activity should be gradually increased as their pain allows (grade of recommendation: A). Some people may require work or lifting restrictions at the discretion of the physician, especially if their job requires heavy lifting.

Once a patient's activity level is established, other lifestyle modifications, such as weight loss, initiation of an exercise program, and tobacco cessation, can be attempted (grade of recommendation: C). These nonmedical therapies do not lend themselves to easy comparison and analysis via randomized, double-blind, placebo-controlled clinical trials. Changing certain lifestyle factors has been shown to help current LBP episodes and to decrease recurrence, but findings vary from study to study [12]. Exercise programs that incorporate aerobic exercise with strengthening of the back can reduce recurrence rates of LBP, but a systematic review states that these results had mixed data, were only conducted in the workplace, had low numbers (total $n < 350$ in 16 studies), and were limited in follow-up (longest study = 18 months) [27]. Lahad et al [27] reported limited evidence to recommend exercises for primary prevention of LBP in asymptomatic individuals and insufficient evidence for recommending other means of prevention, including education and risk factor modification (level of evidence: 2; lower-quality randomized control trial [RCT]). Epidemiologic studies have suggested that there may be a preventive value to weight loss and smoking cessation, but no intervention trials to demonstrate this have been reported [12] (level of evidence: 2; cohort studies).

Exercise and physical therapy are often used to help treat acute, subacute, and chronic back pain. Exercise therapy has not been shown to be more effective for acute back pain (defined as <12 weeks in the analysis) as compared with maintaining usual activity [28,29] (level of evidence: 1; systematic review). Numerous different types of exercises have been applied as treatment for chronic back pain (defined as episodes lasting ≥ 12 weeks). The Cochrane Group [28] evaluated the available literature on several different types of exercises and found inconsistent evidence that exercises can help patients with chronic LBP return to normal daily activities, including work (level of evidence: 1; systematic review). Of the types of exercises studied, no one method was superior, but those with graded activity seemed to do better. Physical therapy does not lend itself to rigorous analysis because "physical therapy" is difficult to define. Physical therapy is highly dependent on patient motivation and is highly operator dependent. In addition, the physical therapy prescription should be individualized to each particular patient. It is our standard practice to use physical therapy liberally in the treatment regimens of LBP patients (grade of recommendation: D).

PHARMACOLOGIC THERAPIES

Analgesics are often used to relieve pain and control an acute attack. Patients often take over-the-counter remedies, such as acetaminophen and ibuprofen, before being instructed to do so by a physician. Nonsteroidal anti-inflammatory drugs (NSAIDs) and acetaminophen are considered the drugs of choice in the management of acute back pain [30] (grade of recommendation: A). The most widely prescribed medications for episodes of acute LBP are NSAIDs [30]. Van Tulder et al [30], writing for the Cochrane Group, reported that patients did better on NSAIDs versus placebo for global improvement after 1 week (pooled relative risk [RR] 1.24, 95% CI 1.10–1.41) and for analgesia (pooled RR 1.29, 95% CI 1.05–1.57) (level of evidence: 1; systematic review). The Cochrane group performing the review stated that the various types of NSAIDs within this class are equally effective for acute back pain [30] (level of evidence: 1; systematic review).

There is limited evidence available comparing NSAIDs to acetaminophen. The Cochrane Collaboration Back Review Group [31] reviewed five studies directly comparing the efficacy of NSAIDs to acetaminophen. Of these, the only high-quality study demonstrated better outcomes in the NSAID-treated group (diflunisal 500 mg bid for 4 weeks; $n = 16$) versus the acetaminophen arm (1000 mg qid for 4 weeks; $n = 13$) in patients with chronic LBP [32]. A study limited by methodologic flaws ($n = 60$) demonstrated a slight, statistically significant benefit of NSAIDs (mefenamic acid 500 mg tid for 1 week) versus acetaminophen (1000 mg qid for 1 week) in acute LBP [33]. In two low-quality studies, there was no difference in outcomes between patients treated with NSAIDs versus acetaminophen [31]. Therefore, there is inconsistent evidence that NSAIDs are more effective than acetaminophen for acute LBP (level of evidence: 3), and the use of acetaminophen is generally not recommended unless NSAIDs are not tolerated (grade of recommendation: B).

We could find no head-to-head studies that demonstrate a statistically significant advantage of COX-2 inhibitors to traditional NSAIDs. Many studies demonstrated equal efficacy of the two medication classes, and the published trials demonstrate a beneficial side-effect profile with regard to gastrointestinal (GI) side effects while maintaining equivalent efficacy. Given the increasing concern over COX-2 inhibitors and cardiovascular (particularly thrombotic) side effects, we recommend the use of traditional NSAIDs for analgesia and do not routinely recommend COX-2 inhibitors for patients with acute LBP (grade of recommendation: B).

Muscle relaxants are another frequently prescribed medication for acute back pain. Cyclobenzaprine and others like it are called muscle relaxants, but it is not clear that there is any activity on the neuromuscular spindle. Instead, the drug acts on the central nervous system to decrease muscular tone [34]. According to a systematic review of patients treated with cyclobenzaprine, patients were nearly five times as likely to report symptom improvement by day 14 compared with patients in the placebo arm (odds ratio 4.7, 95% CI 2.7–8.1, $P = 0.002$), and the number needed to treat to see an improvement was 2.7 (95% CI 2.0–4.2) [35] (level of evidence: 1, systematic review). Although these medicines may seem helpful, the benefit arises at the price of significant side effects, particularly sedation; more than half of the patients in the studies reported experiencing adverse events [35]. The beneficial effect was greatest in the first 4 days, indicating that shorter courses may be better [35].

A Cochrane Database review of muscle relaxants [36] was done to evaluate the literature on the drugs as a class, not limited to only cyclobenzaprine. These medicines have a significant effect versus placebo on short-term (2–4 days) pain relief (RR 0.80, 95% CI 0.71–0.89, $P < 0.05$) and global efficacy (RR 0.49, 95% CI 0.25–0.95, $P < 0.05$) [36] (level of evidence: 1; systematic review). The RR for all adverse events was higher (RR 1.50, 95% CI 1.14–1.98, $P < 0.05$), especially CNS sedation (RR 2.04, 95% CI 1.23–3.37, $P < 0.05$) [36] (level of evidence: 1; systematic review). Although they are often prescribed in conjunction with NSAIDs, there is not necessarily an additive benefit because studies have shown inconsistent results [37]. We believe that muscle relaxants may be helpful in small doses and short courses and that their use should be reserved for patients with bothersome night symptoms (grade of recommendation: B).

Narcotic analgesics are commonly prescribed for acute back pain. Narcotics can be helpful to control episodes of severe or debilitating pain, but liberal use of these medicines must be done with caution. In addition to common side effects of constipation, GI upset, and sedation, patients must be warned of potential dependence. This risk is lower when narcotics are used for short-term treatment. There have not been high-quality, large-scale RCTs comparing narcotics to acetaminophen or NSAIDs. Although several studies have demonstrated the efficacy of narcotics as a medical treatment of last resort, there are limited data on their use in the acute setting. Some physicians feel comfortable prescribing narcotics liberally for acute pain, but we reserve narcotics for the more severe episodes of acute or chronic LBP. If narcotics are used, it is important to also prescribe stool softeners because straining from narcotic-induced constipation can further aggravate LBP [7].

Tramadol, used alone or in combination with acetaminophen, is another choice for acute and chronic LBP. A RCT of tramadol/ acetaminophen versus placebo for the management of LBP ($n = 318$) demonstrated efficacy, and the use of the study medication was discontinued due to insufficient pain relief in only 22% of patients versus 41% for placebo [38] (level of evidence: 1; RCT). This medicine provides another means of achieving analgesia, with fewer side effects than narcotics and less potential for addiction (grade of recommendation: A).

Injection therapies are used to provide local corticosteroid or anesthetics in direct proximity to affected areas in patients with pain or radiculopathy. The injections can be done locally in the epidural space or into the facet joints and have been performed with or without imaging guidance. A systematic review of 21 RCTs of patients with LBP lasting longer than 1 month reported inconsistent results on the effects of injections for LBP [39] (level of evidence: 1; systematic review). A review by Koes et al [40] was complicated by difficulty in comparing different RCTs for epidural steroid injections (ESIs) because the studies were of different design. Of 12 studies reviewed, six showed a benefit. Although flaws in study design precluded better assessment, Koes et al conclude that, although ESIs may be beneficial, it seems that the benefit is short-lived [40] (level of evidence: 2; lower-quality RCTs). Despite the inconsistent evidence, we have found ESI to be a helpful treatment modality in carefully selected patients with acute or subacute discogenic pain (grade of recommendation: D).

OTHER THERAPEUTIC OPTIONS

Patients with LBP may seek spinal manipulation. A review was performed of RCTs that evaluated spinal manipulation versus other therapies, including sham laser, conventional general practitioner care, analgesics, physical therapy, structured exercises, or back school. Spinal manipulation was superior only to sham manipulation therapy (10-mm difference [95% CI 2–17 mm] on a 100-mm visual analog scale), and there was no evidence that it was superior to other treatments for acute or chronic LBP [41] (level of evidence: 1; systematic review). We do not routinely recommend spinal manipulation because it has not been shown to be better than other methods, even though it is generally well tolerated by patients (grade of recommendation: C).

Cherkin et al [42] performed a comparison between chiropractic manipulation, physical therapy (using the McKenzie method), and providing patients with an educational handbook. The results of the study were that manipulation and physical therapy had similar costs and expenses, but the outcomes of chiropractic care were marginally better than the outcomes of receiving an educational booklet. The results at 4 weeks of treatment on an 11-point unvalidated "Bothersome Scale" for each arm of the study (the educational booklet, chiropractic manipulation, or McKenize physical therapy) were 3.1 (95% CI 2.4–3.9), 1.9 (95% CI 1.5–2.2), and 2.3 (95% CI 1.9–2.8), respectively ($P = 0.007$). At 12 weeks, the "bothersomeness of symptoms" on the 11-point scale were 3.2 (95% CI 2.4–4.0), 2.0 (95% CI 1.6–2.4), and 2.7 (95% CI 2.2–3.3), respectively ($P = 0.02$), with lower numbers representing less bothersome symptoms. When the three groups were rated by the Roland Disability Score, there was no statistically significant difference between the groups (level of evidence: 1; high-quality RCT).

Chiropractic manipulation may not have been shown to be more effective than other treatments, but it is still used by many patients with LBP. In a survey of North Carolina residents ($n = 3505$) with LBP, those who went to a chiropractor compared with those who were treated by medical doctors were more likely to feel that the treatment was helpful (99% versus 80%), more likely to be satisfied with the care they received (96% versus 84%), and less likely to seek care from another provider for the same episode of pain (14% versus 27%) [4] (level of evidence: 2; cohort study). Because it has not been shown to be superior to other treatments, we are not routinely in favor of or against chiropractic manipulation for patients with LBP (grade of recommendation: D).

Transcutaneous electrical nerve stimulation (TENS) has been studied for treatment of back pain, although it is used more often in chronic back pain. A meta-analysis of five trials demonstrated no evidence to support the use of TENS for chronic back pain [43]. There was no statistically significant difference between active TENS and placebo TENS for any outcome measure. The review was limited by inconsistent data on the use of the devices due to variation in site of application, duration of treatment, and optimal frequency or intensity to use (level of evidence: 2; systematic review of low-quality RCTs). Therefore, we do not support the routine use of TENS (grade of recommendation: B).

Prolotherapy attempts to treat chronic pain by injection of irritant solutions, a method believed to strengthen weak or damaged ligaments, thereby reducing pain and disability. Yelland et al [44] report inconsistent evidence on the benefits of prolotherapy (level of evidence: 2; systematic review of low-quality RCTs). The use of prolotherapy is not supported by the available medical literature and is not recommended by the authors (grade of recommendation: D). Massage and acupuncture are two other nonmedical therapies often used to treat LBP. Furlan et al [45] performed a systematic review of eight RCTs comparing massage therapy to other modalities and concluded that massage was inferior to manipulation and TENS, equal to corsets and exercises, and superior to relaxation therapy, acupuncture, and self-care education (level of evidence: 1; systematic review). The review stated that different styles of massage have not demonstrated that one is superior to another. The reviewers concluded that massage might be beneficial for patients with subacute and chronic nonspecific LBP. A separate analysis of acupuncture failed to show that it is an effective treatment for back pain compared with other modalities [46]. There is not enough high-quality evidence to warrant the routine recommendation of massage or acupuncture for patients with LBP (grade of recommendation: B).

Back School and other joint protection programs are often prescribed for the treatment of back pain. The original Back School was developed in Sweden in 1980. They have been adopted and modified many times since then. Van Tulder et al [47] reviewed 15 RCTs (only three were considered high quality) to determine the impact Back Schools had on pain. The results indicated that there is moderate evidence that Back Schools have better short-term effects compared with placebo or waiting list controls. The reviewers concluded that Back Schools may be effective for patients with recurrent and chronic LBP, but cost effectiveness could not be determined because the results were mixed. A more recently updated Cochrane review concluded that "there is moderate evidence suggesting that back schools, in an occupational setting, reduce pain, and improve function and return-to-work status, in the short and intermediate-term, compared with exercises, manipulation, myofascial therapy, advice, placebo or waiting list controls, for patients with chronic and recurrent LBP," but numerical data were unavailable [48]. We reserve the use of Back Schools for patients with subacute or chronic pain that interferes with the ability to work (grade of recommendation: B).

Heat and ice therapies are used frequently. Heat is thought to relieve pain, and ice is believed to decrease swelling. These two therapies subjectively help some patients, but results are inconsistent. The Agency for Health care Research and Quality guidelines found no evidence of its benefit for acute LBP; however, self-application of heat or cold to temporarily relieve symptoms has been recommended by other authors due to low cost and noninvasiveness [7,12] (level of evidence: 3; consensus guideline). Given the minimal cost and noninvasiveness of these methods, it is reasonable to recommend a trial to see if there is any improvement, but it should not be the only therapy offered (grade of recommendation: D).

SURGICAL TREATMENT OPTIONS

Surgery for acute back pain is rare. Only a minority of patients with chronic back pain require surgical intervention. Patients with severe neurologic compromise, such as cord compression or cauda equina syndrome, should undergo surgical decompression or discectomy. Surgery may be considered if all four of the following criteria are met in the presence of progressive neurologic deficits: (1) leg pain $\geq$ back pain, (2) positive SLR, (3) no response to nonsurgical therapy for 4 to 6 weeks for herniated disc or 8 to 12 weeks for spinal stenosis, and (4) imaging confirms corresponding lesion [2,49]. Exceptions to the rule are few, but infections such as an epidural abscess may need to be drained operatively, and compression fractures or an unstable vertebral column may need hardware to stabilize the spine. Surgery is used more in patients with severe subacute (>6 weeks) or chronic back pain. Discectomy has also been shown to be an effective treatment for radicular pain due to lumbar disc prolapse in selected patients [50]. Although spinal fusion surgery has been used for numerous reasons most authors feel that the only definite indication for fusion is in patients with unstable spondylolisthesis [51].

Surgery for spinal stenosis is often used to treat patients who fail nonsurgical interventions. In a review of treatments for degenerative lumbar spinal stenosis by Synder et al [52], patients failing nonsurgical treatment had improvement of symptoms after surgery, and the outcomes were better at 4 years follow-up (level of evidence: 2; clinical cohort study). Patients with spinal stenosis, neurogenic claudication, and restricted walking had an increase in time to development of symptoms (mean increase from 2 to 12 minutes) and total ambulation time (mean increase 7 to 13 minutes) (level of evidence: 2; uncontrolled study). Although the improvements in time to first symptoms and total ambulation time are not more than 10 minutes, the increase may make a substantial difference is a patients' quality of life.

Surgical rates and outcomes are highly variable. A study of spinal surgery ($n = 655$) showed that those who underwent surgery in areas with the lowest rate of surgical management had superior outcomes to those operated on in the highest-rate areas [53]. Although discectomies and laminectomies are common procedures, newer surgical options are emerging (eg, lumbar disc replacement).

PROGRESSION TO CHRONIC BACK PAIN

Recurrences of LBP are common. In a follow-up study of primary care patients with a history of LBP ($n = 1128$), 69% to 82% of patients who had back pain in the 12 previous months experienced another episode within 30 days before the survey [6]. Not all chronic back pain comes from acute attacks that never fully healed; recurrent back pain can lead to chronic pain just as easily. Several risk factors have been validated that may help identify a patient at risk to develop persistent symptoms, including history of back pain, depression, psychologic distress, substance abuse, pending or past litigation, or disability compensation regarding the injury, low socioeconomic status, and work dissatisfaction [2].

Waddell et al [54] initially described a series of physical examination findings that are consistent with poor response to traditional treatment. The "Waddell signs" include inconsistencies on seated versus supine SLR testing, superficial or widespread tenderness, sensory or motor findings inconsistent with anatomic distribution (eg, stocking distribution of neurologic findings versus dermatomal), pain with axial loading (pressing down on top of head), and general over-reaction during the examination. It is uncertain whether earlier identification of patients at higher risk of treatment failure helps to prevent the treatment failure. Some authors suggest that earlier referral for physical or cognitive-behavioral therapy may be of benefit in these high-risk patients [55].

For patients with chronic LBP, several types of medicines from many different classes are used to try to achieve some degree of analgesia.

Among these are long-acting narcotics, anti-seizure medicines, topical creams and anesthetics, and antidepressants. The primary goal in the treatment of patients with chronic LBP is to reduce symptoms to a level that is tolerable and to help the patient achieve a satisfactory level of functioning. It is often unrealistic to expect the patient to be completely pain free.

SUMMARY

The majority of LBP is benign and can be treated with nonsurgical methods. The mainstays of therapy are continuing activity within limits of pain, lifestyle modification, analgesic and anti-inflammatory medicine, and supportive care. Red flags that should alarm providers include severe or progressive pain in patients over 50 years of age, history of malignancy, fevers, night symptoms, or neurologic compromise. These characteristics should prompt further work-up.

Imaging is not necessary in most instances. Plain films can be used to evaluate for osseous lesion or fracture, and MRI can be used to evaluate for degenerative disc disease, herniated discs, and spinal stenosis. A surgical evaluation should be obtained for any patient with possible cauda equine or cord compression (symptoms of saddle anesthesia, urinary dysfunction) or when conservative management fails.

References

[1] Andersson G. Epidemiological features of chronic low back pain. Lancet 1999;354:581–5.
[2] Atlas SJ, Deyo RA. Evaluating and managing acute low back pain in the primary care setting. J Gen Intern Med 2001;16:120–31.
[3] Jarvik J, Deyo R. Diagnostic evaluation of low back pain with emphasis on imaging. Ann Intern Med 2002;137:586–95.
[4] Carey TS, Evans AT, Hadler NM, et al. Acute severe low back pain: a population-based study of prevalence and care seeking. Spine 1996;21:339–44.
[5] Carey TS, Garrett JM, Jackman A, et al. The outcomes and costs of care for acute low back pain among patients seen by primary care practitioners, chiropractors, and orthopedic surgeons. N Engl J Med 1995;333:913–8.
[6] Von Korff M, Deyo RA, Cherkin DC, et al. Back pain in primary care: outcomes at 1 year. Spine 1993;18:855–62.
[7] Lehrich JR, Sheon RP. Treatment of low back pain: initial approach. UpToDate 2004;12. Available at: http://www.utdol.com/application/topic.asp?file=spinaldi/4659. Accessed April 22, 2005.
[8] Pengel H, Maher C, Refshauge K. Systematic review of conservative interventions for subacute low back pain. Clin Rehabil 2002;16:811–20.
[9] Deyo RA, Rainville J, Kent DL. What can the history and physical examination tell us about low back pain? JAMA 1992;268:760–5.
[10] Van der Linden S, van der Heijde D. Ankylosing spondylitis: clinical features. Rheum Dis Clin North Am 1998;24:663–76.
[11] Deyo R, Tsui-Wu Y-J. Descriptive epidemiology of low-back pain and its related medical care in the United States. Spine 1987;12:264–8.
[12] Deyo RA, Weinstein JN. Primary care: low back pain. N Engl J Med 2001;344:363–70.
[13] Coste J, Delecoeuillerie G, Cohen de Lara A, et al. Clinical course and prognostic factors in acute low back pain: an inception cohort study in primary care practice. BMJ 1994;308:577–80.

[14] Lehrich JR, Katz JN, Sheon RP. Approach to the diagnosis and evaluation of low back pain in adults. UpToDate 2004;12. Available at: http://www.utdol.com/application/topic.asp?file=spinaldi/2946. Accessed April 22, 2005.

[15] Garry J, McShane J. Lumbar spondylolysis in adolescent athletes. J Fam Pract 1998;47: 145–9.

[16] Xin S, Zhang Q, Fan D. Significance of the straight-leg-raising test in the diagnosis and clinical evaluation of lower lumbar intervertebral-disc protrusion. J Bone Joint Surg 1987;69:517–22.

[17] Jonsson B, Stromqvist B. Symptoms and signs of degeneration of the lumbar spine. J Bone Joint Surg 1993;75:381–5.

[18] Netter FH. Atlas of human anatomy. 2nd edition. East Hanover (NJ): Novartis; 1997.

[19] Carragee E, Kim D, van der Vlugt T, et al. The clinical use of erythrocyte sedimentation rate in pyogenic vertebral osteomyelitis. Spine 1997;22:2089–93.

[20] Lehrich JR, Sheon RP. Laboratory evaluation of low back pain. UpToDate 2004;12. Available at: http://www.utdol.com/application/topic.asp?file=spinaldi/4962. Accessed April 22, 2005.

[21] Jensen M, Brant-Zawadzki M, Obuchiwski N, et al. Magnetic resonance imaging of the lumbar spine in people without back pain. N Engl J Med 1994;331:69–73.

[22] Jarvik J, Hollingworth W, Heagerty P, et al. The Longitudinal Assessment of Imaging and Disability of the Back (LAIDBack) study: baseline data. Spine 2001;26:1158–66.

[23] Borenstein D. The value of magnetic resonance imaging of the lumbar spine to predict low-back pain in asymptomatic subjects. J Bone Joint Surg 2001;83-A:1306–11.

[24] Hagen K. Review: bed rest is not effective for acute low-back pain or sciatica. J Bone Joint Surg 2001;83-A, 789.

[25] Hagen K, Hilde G, Jamtvedt G, et al. Bed rest for acute low-back pain and sciatica. Cochrane Database Syst Rev 2004;4:CD001254.

[26] Hilde G, Hagen K, Jamtvedt G, et al. Advice to stay active as a single treatment for low back pain and sciatica. Cochrane Database Syst Rev 2002;2:CD003632.

[27] Lahad A, Malter AD, Berg AO, et al. The effectiveness of four interventions for the prevention of low back pain. JAMA 1994;272:1286–91.

[28] Van Tulder M, Malmivaara A, Esmail R, et al. Exercise therapy for low back pain. Spine 2000;25:2784–96.

[29] Faas A. Exercises: which ones are worth trying, for which patients, and when? Spine 1996;21:2874–9.

[30] Van Tulder M, Schikten R, Koes B, et al. Non-steroidal anti-inflammatory drugs for low-back pain. Cochrane Database Syst Rev 2004;2.

[31] Van Tulder M, Maurits W, Scholten R, et al. Nonsteroidal anti-inflammatory drugs for low back pain: a systematic review within the framework of the Cochrane Collaboration Back Review Group. Spine 2000;25:2501–13.

[32] Hickey R. A comparison of diflunisal with paracetamol. N Z Med J 1982;95:312–4.

[33] Evans D, Burke M, Newcombe R. Medicines of choice in low back pain. Curr Med Res Opin 1980;6:540–7.

[34] Fischer JD. Drugdex Drug Evaluations: Cyclobenzaprine. Micromedix. Available at: http://www.thomsonhc.com/hcs/librarian/PFPUI/un45xHtJ1UCcD/ND_PG/PRIH/CS/D00E4F/ND_T/HCS/ND_P/Main/DUPLICATIONSHIELDSYNC/071826/ND_B/HCS/PFActionld/hcs.main.FollowLink/cgiexe/:mdxcgi:display.exe/scid/41053145/cgiparm/CTL=:production:ocmcontent:ocmcontent:20_Q1:mdxcgi:MEGAT.SYS&SET=426942 C42EF860&SYS=1&T=526&M=80299. Accessed December 6, 2004.

[35] Browning R, Jackson J, O'Malley P. Cyclobenzaprine and back pain: a meta-analysis. Arch Intern Med 2001;161:1613–20.

[36] Van Tulder M, Touray T, Furlan AD, et al. Muscle relaxants for non-specific low back pain. Cochrane Database Syst Rev 2003;2:CD004252.

[37] Turturro M, Frater C, D'Amico F. Cyclobenzaprine with ibuprofen versus ibuprofen alone in acute myofascial strain. Ann Emerg Med 2003;41:818–26.

[38] Ruoff G, Rosenthal N, Jordan D, et al. Tramadol/acetaminophen combination tablets for the treatment of chronic lower back pain: a multicenter, randomized, double-blind, placebo-controlled outpatient study. Clin Ther 2003;25:1123–41.

[39] Nelemans P, de Bie R, de Vet H, et al. Injection therapy for subacute and chronic benign low-back pain. Cochrane Database Syst Rev 2000;2:CD001824.

[40] Koes BW, Scholten R, Mens J, et al. Efficacy of epidural steroid injections for low-back pain and sciatica: a systematic review of randomized clinical trials. Pain 1995;63:279–88.

[41] Assendelft W, Morton S, Yu E, et al. Spinal manipulative therapy for low back pain. Cochrane Database Syst Rev 2004;1:CD000447.

[42] Cherkin DC, Deyo RA, Battie M, et al. A comparison of physical therapy, chiropractic manipulation, and provision of an educational booklet for the treatment of patients with low back pain. N Engl J Med 1998;339:1021–9.

[43] Milne S, Welch V, Brosseau L, et al. Transcutaneous electrical nerve stimulation (TENS) for chronic low-back pain. Cochrane Database Syst Rev 2001;2:CD003008.

[44] Yelland M, Del Mar C, Pirozzo S, et al. Prolotherapy injections for chronic low-back pain. Cochrane Database Syst Rev 2004;2.

[45] Furlan A, Brosseau L, Imamura M, et al. Massage for low-back pain. Cochrane Database Syst Rev 2002;2:CD001929.

[46] Van Tulder MW, Cherkin D, Berman B, et al. Acupuncture for low-back pain. Cochrane Database Syst Rev 2004;2.

[47] Van Tulder M, Esmail R, Bombardier C, et al. Back schools for non-specific low-back pain. Cochrane Database Syst Rev 2000;2:CD000261.

[48] Heymans M, Van Tulder M, Esmail R, et al. Back schools for non-specific low-back pain. Cochrane Database Syst Rev 2004;4:CD000261.

[49] Lehrich JR, Sheon RP. Treatment of chronic low back pain. Wellesley, MA: UpToDate 2004;12.

[50] Gibson J, Grant I, Waddell G. Surgery for lumbar disc prolapse. Cochrane Database Syst Rev 2000;3:CD001350.

[51] Deyo RA, Nachemson A, Mirza SK. Spinal-fusion surgery: the case for restraint. N Engl J Med 2004;350:722–6.

[52] Snyder D, Doggett D, Turkelson C. Treatment of degenerative lumbar spinal stenosis. Am Fam Physician 2004;70:517–20.

[53] Keller RB, Atlas SJ, Soule DN, et al. Relationship between rates and outcomes of operative treatment for lumbar disc herniation and spinal stenosis. J Bone Joint Surg 1999;81-A:752–62.

[54] Waddell G, McCulloch J, Kummel E, et al. Nonorganic physical signs in low back pain. Spine 1980;5:117–25.

[55] Van Tulder M, Ostelo R, Vlaeyen J, et al. Behavioural treatment for chronic low-back pain. Cochrane Database Syst Rev 2000;2:CD002014.

Address reprint requests to

Marc I. Harwood, MD
Department of Family Medicine
Jefferson Medical College, Thomas Jefferson University
1015 Walnut St, Suite 401
Philadelphia, PA 19107

e-mail: marc.harwood@jefferson.edu

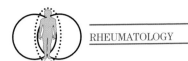
APPROACH TO THE PATIENT WITH ACUTE SWOLLEN/PAINFUL JOINT

Heather Bittner Fagan, MD

In evaluating the patient with an acute swollen painful joint, the clinician must depend on history, physical examination, and appropriate testing to determine the etiology and to direct prompt and effective treatment. The goal in the initial encounter of a patient with joint pain is to determine whether a patient's complaint is intra-articular (ie, within the joint) or extra-articular, inflammatory or noninflammatory, acute or chronic, and localized or widespread [1]. Intra-articular structures include the bone, joint space, cartilage, and intra-articular ligaments. Extra-articular structures include tendons, ligaments, bursa, muscles, nerves, and overlying skin. Arthritis is inflammation of a joint; arthralgia is pain in a joint without inflammation. Arthritis is characterized by the signs of inflammation, warmth, tenderness, erythema, and swelling or effusion. The number of joints involved is an important guide to the clinician. Monoarthritis (inflammation of a single joint) or oligoarthritis (inflammation of a few joints) should be distinguished from polyarthritis. Although there is some similarity in the pathogenesis and prognosis of polyarthritis and oligoarthritis/monoarthritis, the approach to the patient with polyarticular joint pain is different from the approach to the patient with monarticular or oligoarticular joint pain. The etiology of polyarticular joint disease is more likely to be rheumatoid, spondyloarthropathy, or self-limiting [2], whereas monoarticular disease (especially monarthritis) should be regarded as infectious until proven otherwise.

Infection is a relatively common cause of acute joint pain and should be given primary consideration. Infectious arthritis requires prompt

From the Department of Family and Community Medicine, Christiana Care Health System, Wilmington, Delaware; and the Department of Family Medicine, Thomas Jefferson University, Philadelphia, Pennsylvania treatment to prevent joint destruction and spread of infection. This article focuses on monarticular and oligoarticular disease and the similarity of the diagnostic approaches. Although much of this information is pertinent to polyarticular disease, polyarticular joint pain is best reviewed as a separate topic.

CAUSES

Joint pain is associated with a long list of medical disorders (Box 1). Potentially any of these disorders might present as an acute swollen/painful joint. Although most of these etiologies have classic presentations as polyarticular disease or monoarticular disease, there is substantial overlap in the manner of presentation. For example, any polyarticular disease, such as rheumatoid arthritis or systemic lupus erythematosus, can

---

Box 1. Etiology of Joint Pain [6,15,20,24,33]

Infectious
- Bacterial (Table 1)
- Viral (Table 2)
- Fungal
- Reactive/post-infectious (Chlamydia, Streptococcal, Salmonella, Shigella, Yersinia)

Crystalline
- Gout (hyperuricemia)
- Other crystal deposition diseases (pseudogout, a.k.a. calcium pyrophosphate dihydrate deposition disease; hydroxyapatite crystal deposition disease)

Systemic
- Autoimmune (rheumatoid arthritis, systemic lupus erythematosus, juvenile rheumatoid arthritis, mixed connective tissue disease, Behcet syndrome, sarcoidosis)
- Spondyloarthropathy (psoriatic arthritis, ankylosing spondylarthritis, inflammatory bowel disease, Reiter syndrome)
- Vasculitis (Henoch-Schönlein purpura, vasculitis, polyarteritis nodosa, Wegener granulomatosis, giant cell arteritis)
- Malignancy
- Endocrine (hypothyroidism, hypoparathyroidism)

Trauma
- General
- Hemarthrosis
- Iatrogenic (synthetic hyaluronic injection, drug reactions [penicillin])

Other
- Fibromyalgia
- Depression

initially present in a single joint and later be revealed to occur in other joints. Therefore, the clinician must consider a broad number of possible causes in approaching the patient with the acute swollen or painful joint.

The etiology of most joint pain can be broadly divided into infectious, crystalline, systemic, and traumatic. Infectious etiologies may encompass acute infections (bacterial, viral, and infrequently fungal), chronic infections, and reactive or postinfectious etiologies. Systemic etiologies include autoimmune pathologies and spondyloarthropathies, vasculitis, malignancy, endocrine disorders, and others. Traumatic causes include derangements of the bone and soft tissues and are often associated with an effusion.

Certain etiologies are more common in monoarticular joint disease and should be given primary consideration (Box 2). The acute, swollen/painful joint is most commonly caused by trauma, infection, or crystal-related disease. Trauma is the most common cause, followed by infection [3]. Gout, the most common crystal-associated arthropathy, is a common cause of the acute swollen, painful joint [4].

Musculoskeletal Infections

Infection can occur in any musculoskeletal structure. Infection of the joint space (infectious arthritis), bone (osteomyelitis), and bursa are the most common [5]. Of these infections, infectious arthritis is the most common consideration in the patient with an acute painful, swollen joint.

Acute Bacterial Arthritis

Acute bacterial arthritis, or septic arthritis, is a medical emergency due to the possibility or joint destruction and mortality [5,6]. Bacteria generally gain access to the sterile joint space through hematologic spread. Other mechanisms are proposed in certain infectious diseases; for example, immune complex formation is the likely pathogenesis in bacterial endocarditis and disseminated gonococcal infection. Inflammation and inflammatory cytokines are considered to be the primary mechanism of joint damage. The classic picture of a red, hot, swollen joint with systemic symptoms and elevated serum white blood cell count has been cited to

---

Box 2. Common Etiology of Acute Monoarticular Joint Pain

- Trauma—Most common (90%) [3]
- Nongonococcal infection—*Staphylococcus aureus* most common
- Gonococcal infection—Most common after S aureus[a]
- Gout and other crystal deposition

[a]Sources differ on whether *Neisseria gonorrhoeae* or *S aureus* is more common; this is probably due to differences in populations studied [5,19].

occur in 70% to 80% of cases [5]. Most acute bacterial arthritis is monoarthritis, but polyarticular infectious arthritis occurs in about 12% to 20% of cases, depending on the population considered [5].

The infectious etiology varies according to patient factors, particularly age and sexual activity [6,7]. *Staphylococcus aureus* is cited as the most common cause of infectious monoarthritis in adults [5,7]. *Neisseria gonorrhea*, a sexually transmitted organism, is the most common cause of acute monoarthritis in young, sexually active adults. A wide variety of pathogens can cause acute infectious arthritis, and these are listed according to Gram stain characteristics in Table 1.

Pediatric musculoskeletal infections and infectious arthritis have different considerations from adult infectious arthritis and are not reviewed fully here. Neonates and children are at higher risk for group B streptococcus, *S aureus*, *Escherichia coli*, and other Gram-negative organisms. *Haemophilus influenza* used to be a common joint pathogen in young children before effective vaccination. *S aureus* and *E coli* have become more dominant pathogens in this group.

TABLE 1.
Causes of Bacterial Arthritis Organized by Gram Stain Characteristics

Gram-positive organisms	
Cocci	***Staphylococcus aureus***[a]
	S epidermidis
	Streptococcus pyogenes,
	S pneumoniae, ***S viridans*, other**
	B-hemolytic including Group B and G
	Peptococcus, Peptostreptococcus
Rods	*Listeria monocytogenes*
	Corynebacterium pyogenes
	Clostridium
Gram-negative organisms	
Cocci	***Neisseria gonorrhoeae***
	N meningitidis
	Moraxella
Rods	***Escherichia coli*, Pseudomonas**,
	Haemophilus influenza, Klebsiella,
	Pasteurella, Proteus, Brucella,
	Campylobacter, Salmonella, Serratia,
	Bacteroides, Fusobacterium
Indeterminate staining	
Spirochetes[b]	*Borrelia burgdorferi*
	Treponema pallidum
Mycoplasma	*Mycoplasma hominis*
	M pneumoniae
	Ureaplasma urealyticum

[a] More common in bold.
[b] Gram-negative but not usually visible by light microscopy due to size.

In adults, acute bacterial arthritis is generally divided into nongonococcal and gonococcal. The clinician must consider nongonococcal disease in older patients and in patients without a history of possible gonorrheal exposure. In contrast to gonococcal infections, nongonococcal infections (eg, *S aureus*) tend to occur in joints with some abnormality. Risk factors for septic joint include skin infection, prosthetic joint, joint surgery, rheumatoid arthritis, age greater than 80 years, and diabetes [7,8]. Acquired or congenital immunosuppression and other comorbidities are likely risk factors [5]. Coexisting conditions can place patients at increased risk for infectious arthritis and can predispose patients to infection in less common joints and with less common pathogens. For instance, intravenous drug use allows organisms to bypass the innate immune system and to access joints, such as the sternoclavicular joint, uncommonly thought of in infectious arthritis. In individuals with indwelling catheters, organisms with low pathogenicity, such as Pseudomonas, can establish infection. Sickle cell disease is associated with *Salmonella* infections.

Disseminated gonococcal infection is a common cause of infectious arthritis in the young, sexually active adult. This arthritic stage of disease is often preceded by an asymptomatic genitourinary infection and a transient bacteremia.

Tuberculosis

Tuberculosis can present as an acutely painful swollen joint. Mycobacterial infections are generally thought to occur slowly and indolently. In presumed infectious arthritis in immunocompromised hosts or in cases that seem to be refractory to standard antibiotic therapy, the clinician should consider *Mycobacterium tuberculosis* and other uncommon pathogens, including mycoplasma.

Lyme Disease

Lyme disease, infection with *Borrelia burgdorferi*, is rare etiology of acute monoarthritis occurring in endemic areas. A history of rash consistent with erythema migrans or tick exposure suggests Lyme disease. Lyme disease presents with acute monoarthritis in 10% of cases [6] and often requires serologic testing for confirmation.

Viral Arthritis

Viral arthritis is also a consideration (Table 2). Although a large number of viruses can cause oligo- or monoarthritis, viruses more commonly associated with this presentation include Hepatitis B, HIV, parvovirus B19, and rubella [5,9,10].

Fungal Arthritis

Another uncommon cause of infectious arthritis is fungal infection. Fungal infections should be considered in older individuals, in

TABLE 2.
Viral Etiologies of Acute Monoarthritis

Parvovirus B19	Fifths disease or erythema infectiosum
Infectious Hepatitis	A, B or C but B is most common
HIV	
HTLV-1	
EBV	
Measles, mumps, **rubella**	
Adenovirus	
VZV	
Alpha viruses	Uncommon in the United States
*more common in **bold**	

immunocompromised individuals, and in patients with indwelling catheters. Candidal infections can be acute and involve a single joint. However, most fungal infections are thought to occur slowly and indolently in one or a few joints. Fungal infections should be suspected in cases of suspected infectious arthritis that is refractory to standard antibiotic treatment.

Polyarticular Septic Arthritis

Polyarticular septic arthritis accounts for 12% to 20% of septic arthritis. It is more likely to occur in elderly patients and in patients with rheumatoid arthritis and has a higher associated mortality [5].

Prosthetic and Surgical Infections

Surgical history is important in the evaluation of the patient with acute monoarthritis. Recent surgery and joint prosthesis are risk factors for acute infectious monoarthritis. Acute monoarthritis in these patients requires prompt attention and orthopedic referral. Infection of a prosthesis is typically seeded from a skin wound, so wound culture can be helpful. Most infections are considered early infections, occurring within the first 6 months after transplant. Loosening of the prosthesis can cause acute pain and can be confused with infection.

Reactive Arthritis

Group A streptococcal pharyngitis can be associated with a post-streptococcal arthritis, especially in children and sometimes in adolescents and young adults.

Reiter disease, a pentad of urethritis, conjunctivitis, arthritis, balanitis, and keratoderma blennorrhagica, is often attributed to previous infection with chlamydia, but no definitive etiologic agent has been identified. Shigella, Salmonella, and Yersinia infections have been associated with postinfectious arthritis [11].

Crystal-Induced Arthropathies

These diseases can be intra-articular or extra-articular and can be acute or chronic. Due to the inflammatory nature or crystal deposition, these diseases often present as the acute, painful swollen joint [12,13].

Gout

Gout, the deposition of monosodium urate crystals, is the most common crystal-associated disease and presents in a monoarticular fashion in 80% of cases [6]. Although gout can affect almost any joint, the classic presentation of gout is in the first metatarsophalangeal joint, followed by the ankle, midfoot, or knee. Gout and pseudogout and other crystal deposition disease can present with abrupt onset on pain and effusion, raising the suspicion of infection.

Pseudogout

Pseudogout, the deposition of calcium pyrophosphate, is difficult to distinguish clinically from gout and also commonly presents as acute monoarthritis with effusion.

Other Crystal Deposition Diseases

Other crystal deposition diseases include oxalate gout and hydroxyapatite deposition.

Trauma

Trauma is the most common cause of acute monoarthritis. Trauma includes a long differential diagnosis. Intra-articular trauma is more likely than extra-articular trauma to present as acute monoarthritis; fracture, meniscal tears, and other internal derangements (eg, ligament tears) are common forms of intra-articular trauma. The presence of bone marrow elements (eg, fat droplets) in synovial fluid suggests intra-articular trauma.

The history of trauma is a potential pitfall in the approach to the patient with acute monoarthritis. Although some patients with a traumatic etiology may be unable to recall the event, others falsely and inadvertently attribute their joint pain to a relatively minor injury. In a patient with a long-standing history of joint problems, a relatively minor injury can precipitate significant joint pathology, but the history of this injury may be absent from the patient's recalled history. Clinically, the physical examination of a patient with traumatic acute monoarthritis may be indistinguishable from crystal deposition and infectious disease. In fact, trauma can be the precipitant of crystal deposition and infection.

Hemarthrosis, defined as the extravasation of blood into the joint or synovium, indicates trauma. Hemarthrosis must be distinguished from a traumatic tap of the affected joint. Synovial fluid that is consistently bloody or discolored throughout the process of withdrawal and does not clot suggests hemarthrosis. Synovial fluid that is initially clear or yellowish and turns bloody suggests a traumatic arthrocentesis. Hemarthrosis can indicate trauma or a clotting disorder, especially in younger patients.

APPROACH TO THE PATIENT/DIAGNOSIS

History, physical examination, and synovial fluid analysis are the vital components of diagnosis of the acute swollen/painful joint. Prompt evaluation of monoarticular arthritis is crucial because infection must be quickly ruled out to avoid joint destruction.

History

The onset of symptoms is a key determinant in diagnosis. A clear history of abrupt pain occurring seconds to minutes after an injury suggests trauma, including internal derangements, loose body, or fracture. Patients with osteoporosis or long-standing arthritis may present with significant findings but may have a history of a relatively minor injury.

Similar to trauma, infections occur quickly, but the course is less abrupt. In bacterial infection, onset is more likely to be hours to a few days, and in atypical infections (eg, osteomyelitis and fungal infections) onset is slower, occurring over several days to a few weeks. Crystal-associated diseases (eg, gout) can occur over a few hours to a few days but may be distinguished by a history of previous recurrent episodes. An acute exacerbation of chronic joint pain should raise some consideration of a superimposed infection. Rheumatic arthritis is a risk factor for septic arthritis [8].

Other historical symptoms can help imply inflammation or systemic disease. Fever can be an important warning sign of infection. Most patients with an infected joint report a fever at some point during the course of their illness, although they may not appear systemically ill or toxic [4]. High-grade fever is especially concerning, whereas low-grade or remote history of fever may be more of a clue to an autoimmune process. Elderly or immunocompromised patients may fail to mount a fever. General malaise and rash are also associated with infection and autoimmune etiologies. Recent sexual or gastrointestinal infection may precede reactive arthritis.

Information regarding tick bites, joint surgery or replacement, and associated systemic illness guides the clinical approach. Numbness, paraesthesia, or burning may suggest nonarticular disease, such as a myelopathy or neuropathy.

A history of trauma should be obtained, although the history of trauma does not negate the possibility of other etiologies, such as infection and crystal associated disease.

Physical Examination

Careful physical examination allows the clinician to narrow the anatomic source of pain. The physical examination is crucial in determining the localization of pain (ie, intra-articular versus extra-articular) and the presence or absence of inflammation. The physical examination can confirm the history of single-joint involvement and can give clues to any chronic joint condition and systemic illness.

The physical examination, inspection, and palpation can help the clinician to determine an intra-articular versus extra-articular localization of pain. The presence of an effusion and pain are reliable indicators that the process is intra-articular rather than periarticular [11]. Range of motion (ROM) also helps direct the diagnosis. Pain that is roughly equal with active and passive ROM suggests an intra-articular process. Decreased pain with passive ROM compared with active ROM suggests an extra-articular process. Crepitus, locking, deformity, and instability are associated with intra-articular joint pathology.

The examiner should look for the cardinal signs of inflammation; swelling or effusions, erythema or redness, warmth, and tenderness. Swelling or effusions may be obvious but may need to be elicited through ballottement techniques.

Pain directly over the periosteal structures, specifically if the history indicates chronic pain or pain with weight bearing, may represent bone pain and may suggest certain etiologies, such as osteomyelitis and cancer (eg, Paget's disease).

Testing

Synovial fluid aspiration for Gram stain, culture, and other testing is universally recommended in the patient with acute monoarthritis or in other scenarios where infectious arthritis is suspected [3,4,6,7,11,14–20]. There is no evidence for using a particular historical sign or physical symptom to rule in or out the diagnosis of septic joint. Therefore, clinical suspicion of infection warrants synovial fluid testing (grade of recommendation: D; level of evidence: 5).

Briefly, arthrocentesis is typically done by identifying the joint line and penetrating the synovial cavity under sterile conditions. Most joints are easily accessed in the office setting. Some joints, like the hip, may need to be accessed under radiologic guidance. A small amount of synovial fluid is withdrawn for analysis. Procedural details are covered elsewhere [21].

There is debate as to what tests should be ordered for synovial fluid analysis. Conventional wisdom favors a wide approach whereby testing is limited only by the availability of fluid for analysis. However, a large number of commonly ordered tests have limited utility.

Synovial fluid Gram staining and culture are almost universally recommended [5,22]. In nongonococcal septic arthritis, Schmerling [23] estimates the sensitivity of Gram stain to be 50% to 75% and culture to be

75% to 95%; the specificity of Gram stain is reported as "90 plus," and for culture it is reported as "quite high." Samuelson [24] cited that the Gram stain is positive in 50% to 70% of cases, and Weinstein [5] cited that synovial fluid cultures are positive in 70% of cases. A positive culture is a good predictor of septic arthritis. Based on this, the clinician should get a Gram stain and culture of synovial fluid in the acute swollen and painful joint (grade of recommendation: C; level of evidence: 4). Neither a Gram stain nor culture alone has sufficient sensitivity to rule out infection. Therefore, the physician should treat empirically if the clinical scenario strongly suggests infection despite a negative culture or Gram stain (grade of recommendation: C; level of evidence: 4). There is no evidence to support the need for enhanced collection techniques (eg, the collection of synovial fluid in a blood culture container) (grade of recommendation: B; level of evidence: 2b) [25].

Although synovial fluid leukocytosis is an imperfect test that is subject to laboratory variation, it probably has the best clinical utility in predicting inflammatory (and therefore infectious) joint disease [5,16,19,26–28]. Schmerling et al [29] used a synovial white blood cell (WBC) count of <2000 WBC/mm^3 (or 2×10^9 L) to estimate a sensitivity and specificity for predicting inflammatory disease of 0.84% and 0.84%. Septic arthritis was included as a subset of inflammatory arthritis and was not analyzed separately. Weinstein [5] cites that approximately 10% of patients with infection have counts <25,000 WBC/mm^3. In a case review of 50 patients with septic arthritis, none had synovial fluid counts of <2500 WBC/mm^3 [29]. A WBC count of <2000 WBC/mm^3 (or 2×10^9 L) likely has a good negative predictive value for inflammation and, by inference, for infection. Therefore, when the clinical picture does not suggest infection and the WBC count is <2000 WBC/mm^3, empiric antibiotic treatment is not necessary (grade of recommendation: B; level of evidence: 2b). These authors site adequate sensitivity and specificity for percentage of polymorphonuclear cells (PMNs). The presence of >75% PMNs is 75% sensitive and 92% specific for inflammation. Thus, the presence of >75% PMNs has a good positive predictive value for inflammation/infection and should be treated as infection (grade of recommendation: B; level of evidence: 2b). In contrast, these authors found that synovial fluid glucose was not discriminatory.

In addition, synovial fluid leukocytosis of ≥50,000 WBC/mm^3 is used to positively predict infection. Authors cite that counts ≥50,000 WBC/mm^3 occur in 70% of patients with infection [5,29]. Thus, it seems that counts ≥50,000 WBC/mm^3 have good positive predictive value for infection. However, this value of leukocytosis does not have a strong negative predictive value for infection (ie, it cannot be used as a cut-off, and counts lower than 50,000 WBC/mm^3 do not confirm the absence of infection/inflammation). A clinical gap is created in which the clinician has no clear evidence to guide decision making when the count is between 2000 WBC/mm^3 and 50,000 WBC/mm^3. Clinical judgment predominates in this range, with an emphasis on presumptive antibiotic treatment until a diagnosis is established.

In cases of gonococcal disease, mucosal cultures have a higher yield than synovial fluid cultures. Synovial fluid is positive in 50% of cases, whereas mucosal cultures (genital, anal, or oral) are positive in 80% of cases [30]. Thus, in a sexually active patient, all routes of exposure should be cultured (grade of recommendation: B; level of evidence: 2b).

The presence of crystals in synovial fluid is reasonably specific (78% to 99% in pseudogout; 93% to 100% in gout), but sensitivity is variable (56% to 83% in pseudogout; 62.5% to 78% in gout) [28]. Therefore, the presence of crystals "makes the diagnosis," whereas the absence of crystals leaves the clinician dependent on clinical judgment (grade of recommendation: B; level of evidence: 2b).

There is no evidence for or against synovial fluid testing for viral or fungal infections. In suspected Lyme disease, serologic testing, not synovial fluid testing, is recommended [22].

The added utility of blood cultures is unclear. Blood cultures are positive in 50% of cases and likely support diagnosis and treatment in patients with suspected septic arthritis, especially where the synovial fluid culture is negative [5,25].

Other Laboratory Testing

Other serologic tests are adjuncts to care and come into play in specific circumstances, including when other more reliable tests fail to assist the clinician in a diagnostically challenging case [6]. Nonspecific tests (eg, C-reactive protein and erythrocyte sedimentation rate [ESR]) may provide support to a physician's suspicion that disease is inflammatory in nature. An antinuclear antibody test is nonspecific and should be ordered only when a physician has a high suspicion of systemic lupus erythematous or other collaborating evidence for this disease. Likewise, serum rheumatoid factor (RF) is nonspecific and nonsensitive and should be ordered only when the physician has a moderate to high suspicion of disease with corroborating evidence. Other routine blood work should be ordered based on history and physical examination. For example, liver function tests (LFTs) are appropriate when hepatitis is suspected, and coagulation studies are appropriate in the presence of hemarthrosis. Elevated uric acid supports the diagnosis of gout but may be artificially lowered in an acute attack. In the case of an inflamed joint with sterile inflammatory joint fluid, the American College of Rheumatology Ad Hoc Committee recommends a complete blood count, ESR, and RF and recommends considering LFTs, HLA-B27, ANA, Lyme serologies, and pelvic radiograph (grade of recommendation: D; level of evidence: 5).

Radiologic Testing

Other than for trauma and other specific circumstances, radiographs are not usually helpful in the diagnosis of acute swollen and painful joint and should not be routinely obtained. Imaging is recommended by the American College of Rheumatology Ad Hoc Committee when the examination does not localize the anatomic structure causing symptoms, when there is loss of joint function, when pain continues despite appropriate treatment, when a fracture or bone infection is suspected, and when there is a history of malignancy (grade of recommendation: D) [22]. In deep-seated joints like the hip and in special populations like intravenous drug abusers, imaging may help to identify infection. Ultrasound or other imaging may be needed to identify and access a potential septic effusion. Radiologic evaluation of trauma should be guided clinically and may require plain films, computed tomography, and MRI for soft tissue injury. MRI or bone scan (scintography) is indicated in cases of in infiltrative disease, suspected disseminated disease, and osteomyelitis and should be considered in cases of septic joint with inadequate clinical response in 2 to 3 days. An algorithm is presented in Fig. 1 [6,14,16,19,22].

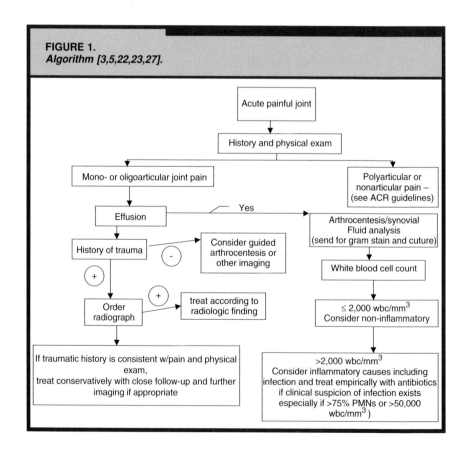

FIGURE 1.
Algorithm [3,5,22,23,27].

TREATMENT

Acute monoarthritis is infectious until proven otherwise. Empiric parenteral antibiotic coverage is required unless the clinician has another likely diagnosis and suspicion for infection is very low. Once a diagnosis is confirmed, the treatment is modified accordingly. The treatment of the acute swollen/painful joint is dependent on the suspected or confirmed etiology.

Infectious Arthritis

Parenteral antibiotics are recommended as treatment for gonococcal and nongonococcal disease [5]. Antibiotic coverage should be aimed at *S aureus* or *N gonorrhea*, depending on the clinical scenario. Taking into consideration the high rate of methicillin resistance in *S aureus*, appropriate choices include beta-lactamase–resistant penicillins, cefazolin, or vancomycin. A third-generation cephalosporin should be used when gonococcal arthritis or Gram-negative organisms are suspected [31]. The spectrum of antibiotic can be narrowed early if a Gram stain result is available. Synovial fluid culture is the most useful in determining antibiotic sensitivity, but a blood culture can guide therapy in cases where infection is suspected and where no synovial fluid pathogen has been isolated.

Although many experts recommend daily aspiration of infected joints or lavage to remove inflammatory products, a Medline search and Cochran search revealed no evidence-based studies addressing this issue. Therefore, this practice is not supported.

Duration of therapy is based on expert opinion and is generally recommended to be 4 weeks or longer in nongonococcal disease. In gonococcal disease, therapy is generally 1 to 2 weeks, and concomitant treatment for chlamydia is recommended for 7 days (grade of recommendation: D; level of evidence: 5).

Surgical drainage of an infected joint is indicated under the following conditions: hip involvement, lack of response to antibiotics, loculation, and suspected anatomic abnormality (grade of recommendation: B; level of evidence: 2b) [17,32].

Trauma

Treatment of the traumatized joint should be tailored to the specific joint and type of injury.

Crystal Deposition Disease

Treatment of gout is divided into acute treatment and long-term management. Acute treatment should aim to reduce pain and inflammation. First-line therapy is a nonsteroidal anti-inflammatory drug (NSAID); indomethacin is the most commonly used NSAID. Colchicine is a common second choice after NSAIDs. Corticosteroids are used when these other agents fail or are contraindicated (grade of recommendation: D; level of evidence: 5). Cochran and Medline do not reveal any large-scale direct comparison trials, so these recommendations are based on safety and cost.

Key Points

- The acute swollen or painful joint should prompt consideration of septic arthritis and necessitates aspiration and synovial fluid analysis.
- The most common causes of the acute swollen or painful joint are trauma, infection, and crystal deposition.
- The history and physical examination are key determinants in the diagnostic algorithm.
- Synovial fluid analysis (specifically, leukocytosis and percentage of PMNs) can indicate the presence or absence of inflammation.
- Ancillary blood testing has a minor role.

References

[1] Cush JJ, Lipsky PE. Approach to articular and musculoskeletal disorders. In: Kasper DL, Fauci AS, Longo DL, et al, editors. Harrison's principles of internal medicine, vol. 311. New York: McGraw Hill; 2005. p. 2028–36.

[2] El-Gabalawy HS, Duray P, Goldbach-Mansky R. Evaluating patients with arthritis of recent onset: studies in pathogenesis and prognosis. JAMA 2000;284:2368–73.

[3] Sack K. Monarthritis: differential diagnosis. Am J Med 1997;102:27.

[4] Baker DG, Schumacher HR Jr. Acute monoarthritis. N Engl J Med 1993;329:1013–20.

[5] Weinstein A, Katz JD. Musculoskeletal infections and crystal-induced arthropathies. In: Lahitta RG, Weinstein A, editors. Educational review manual in rheumatology. 2nd edition. New York: Castle Connolly Graduate Medical Publishing; 2002. p. 1–45.

[6] Helfgott S. Approach to the patient with monarticular joint pain. UptoDate 2005;12:3.

[7] Goldenberg DL. Septic arthritis. Lancet 1998;351:197–202.

[8] Kaandorp CJ, Van Schaardenburg D, Krijnen P, et al. Risk factors for septic arthritis in patients with joint disease: a prospective study. Arthritis Rheum 1995;38:1819–25.

[9] Moore TL. Parvovirus-associated arthritis. Curr Opin Rheumatol 2000;12:289–94.

[10] Ytterberg SR. Viral arthritis. Curr Opin Rheumatol 1999;11:275–80.

[11] Marino CT, Greenwald RA. Acute arthritis. Med Clin North Am 1981;65:177–88.

[12] Meiner SE. Gouty arthritis: not just a big toe problem. Geriatr Nurs (Minneap) 2001;22: 132–4.

[13] Rosenthal AK. Calcium crystal-associated arthritides. Curr Opin Rheumatol 1998;10: 273–7.

[14] Cibere J. Rheumatology: 4. Acute monarthritis. CMAJ 2000;162:1577–83.

[15] Levine M, Siegel LB. A swollen joint: why all the fuss? Am J Ther 2003;10:219–24.

[16] McCune WJ, Golbus J. Monarticular arthritis. In: Ruddy S, editor. Kelley's textbook of rheumatology. 7th edition. Philadelphia: Elsevier; 2005. p. 501–14.

[17] Mikhail IS, Alarcon GS. Nongonococcal bacterial arthritis. Rheum Dis Clin North Am 1993;19:311–31.

[18] Pinals RS. Approach to the patient with polyarticular joint pain. UpToDate 2005;12:3.
[19] Siva C, Velazquez C, Mody A, et al. Diagnosing acute monoarthritis in adults: a practical approach for the family physician. Am Fam Physician 2003;68:83–90.
[20] Till SH, Snaith ML. Assessment, investigation, and management of acute monoarthritis. J Accid Emerg Med 1999;16:355–61.
[21] Zuber TJ. Knee joint aspiration and injection. Am Fam Physician 2002;66:1497–500.
[22] Anonymous. Guidelines for the initial evaluation of the adult patient with acute musculoskeletal symptoms. American College of Rheumatology Ad Hoc Committee on Clinical Guidelines. Arthritis Rheum 1996;39:1–8.
[23] Shmerling RH. Synovial fluid analysis: a critical reappraisal. Rheum Dis Clin North Am 1994;20:503–13.
[24] Samuelson CO, Ward JR. Problems in family practice: joint pain of recent onset. J Fam Pract 1997;5:437–46.
[25] Kortekangas P, Aro H, Lehtonen OP. Synovial fluid culture and blood culture in acute arthritis. Scand J Rheumatol 1995;24:44–7.
[26] Dougados M. Synovial fluid cell analysis. Baillieres Clin Rheumatol 1996;10:519–34.
[27] Shmerling RH, Delbanco TL, Tosteson ANA, et al. Synovial fluid test: what should be ordered? JAMA 1990;264:1009–14.
[28] Swan A, Amer H, Dieppe P. The value of synovial fluid assays in the diagnosis of joint disease: a literature survey. Ann Rheum Dis 2002;61:493–8.
[29] Krey P, Bailen D. Synovial fluid leukocytosis: a study of extremes. Am J Med 1979;67: 436–42.
[30] Cucurull E, Espinoza LR. Gonococcal arthritis. Rheum Dis Clin North Am 1998;24: 305–22.
[31] Wise CM, Morris CR, Wasilauskas BL, et al. Gonococcal arthritis in an era of increasing penicillin resistance: presentations and outcomes in 41 recent cases (1985–1991). Arch Intern Med 1994;154:2690–5.
[32] Broy SB, Schmid FR. A comparison of medical drainage (needle aspiration) and surgical drainage (arthrotomy or arthroscopy) in the initial treatment of infected joints. Clin Rheum Dis 1986;12:501–22.
[33] Bernardeau C, Bucki B, Liote F. Acute arthritis after intra-articular hyaluronate injection: onset of effusions without crystal. Ann Rheum Dis 2001;60:518–20.

Address reprint requests to

Heather Bittner Fagan, MD
1401 Foulk Rd, Ste 100
Family Medicine Center
Wilmington, DE 19803

e-mail: hbittner-fagan@christianacare.org

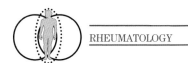
APPROACH TO THE PATIENT WITH RAYNAUD'S PHENOMENON

Dyanne P. Westerberg, DO, and John R. Lawrence, MD

Raynaud's phenomenon is a condition of episodic, reversible, vaso-spastic digital ischemia. It manifests classically as the sequential development of a three-phase color change of blanching, cyanosis, and rubor after cold exposure and subsequent rewarming [1]. In 1862, Maurice Raynaud's described this phenomenon as a localized "syncope." Its duration can vary from a few minutes to hours. It affects the digits in a predictable pattern consistent with previous attacks and is often triggered by cold exposure [2]. Other inciting stimuli, such as emotional stress and trauma, can trigger vasospasm, but historically the threshold to trigger a response is diminished in affected individuals as compared with normal subjects.

DESCRIPTION OF THE THREE-PHASE PHENOMENON

The classic, often well-demarcated, three-phase color change follows the physiologic events of digital arterial vasospasm and its resolution. In phase 1, arterial vasospasm impedes blood flow to the digital capillaries, causing ischemia, visible blanching, and pallor. Paresthesias, numbness, and pain often coincide. In phase 2, the distal capillaries and venules reflexively dilate, pooling with deoxygenated blood and producing cyanosis. With rewarming, the vasospasm resolves and the arteries open, allowing oxygenated blood to flow to the already dilated capillaries and venules, producing the rubor of phase 3. Eventually, vascular tone returns to its normal state, and the digit returns to its baseline color [3]. Although many patients experience the classic three phases of color change, most experience only one or two of the ischemic phases without a hyperemic phase [3].

From the Department of Family and Community Medicine, Christiana Care Health Services, Wilmington, Delaware

EPIDEMIOLOGY

According to the demographic review by Gifford and Hines [4], Raynaud's phenomenon affects women approximately three to five times more frequently than men. It has been described in adults and in children. The average age of onset is 31 years; >75% of patients begin having symptoms before 40 years of age. The onset of symptoms occurs primarily between menarche and menopause. Data on prevalence ranges from 5% to 17%, varying among populations studied according to their location, surrounding climate, time of year, and mean environmental temperature (a larger portion of these individuals reside in colder climates). Duration, frequency, and severity of symptoms increase during the colder months. Although approximately 5% of patients can identify one or more relatives with Raynaud's phenomenon, there is no established genetic predisposition to the idiopathic form of the disorder [4–8]. Other risk factors include cardiovascular disease, low body weight, and advanced age [8].

CLINICAL PRESENTATION AND NATURAL COURSE

Because primary Raynaud's phenomenon is an intermittent series of symptoms in the absence of trophic changes, the presenting physical examination is often normal. The fingers may be cool and may perspire excessively. Radial, ulnar, and pedal pulses should be easily palpable and normal. Sclerodactyly, a thickening and tightening of digital subcutaneous tissues, can develop along with shortening of the distal phalanges, clubbing, and nail deformities [3]. Historically, 40% of patients have progressive involvement of the toes, with only 1% to 2% having isolated toe involvement. In rare cases, the earlobes, tip of the nose, and tongue are involved [3]. Often, the diagnosis must be made by history, the exclusion of secondary conditions, and absence of their typical stigmata.

Although primary idiopathic Raynaud's phenomenon is the most benign form of the disorder, its natural history is not without complications. In the observational study by Gifford and Hines [4], which followed patients over an average of 12 years, 16% reported worsening symptoms, 38% reported no change, 36% reported improvement, and 10% reported complete resolution of symptoms. Sclerodactyly and trophic changes occurred in approximately 10%, with <1% losing part of a digit. Some patients who hold the diagnosis of primary Raynaud's disease for over 20 years may develop scleroderma or other connective tissue disease [4].

PATHOPHYSIOLOGY

Normal regulation of peripheral blood flow depends on several factors, including intrinsic vascular tone, sympathetic nervous activity, circulating neurohumoral substances, and blood viscosity. Although the underlying cause of vasospasm in Raynaud's phenomenon has not been fully elucidated, a combination of various physiologic and pathologic processes have been proposed, supported, and scrutinized in the literature. Proposed functional derangements of increased sympathetic activity, elevated levels of vasoconstrictor hormones, and the influence of exogenous medications have been investigated.

Raynaud originally proposed increased sympathetic nervous system activity as the underlying pathophysiology due to the bilateral and symmetric clinical presentation [2]. Conflicting data from studies of epinephrine concentrations and vasoconstrictor response have not overwhelmingly supported this hypothesis [9–11].

A complimentary hypothesis of local vascular hyper-reactivity to sympathetic stimuli has shown promise in explaining the underlying pathophysiology. A series of studies in human and nonhuman trials has demonstrated that the augmentation of adrenergic-mediated vasoconstriction by cooling occurs despite depression of the contractile machinery or diminished norepinephrine release [12–17]. An increased sensitivity and upregulation of $\alpha2$ receptors with a relative depression of $\alpha1$-receptor activity in response to cold stimuli leads to an exaggerated vasoconstrictor response with exposure to norepinephrine [17,18].

In conditions such as cryoglobulinemia and cold agglutinin disease, it has been well established that hyperviscosity contributes to the overall ischemic and cyanotic phases of Raynaud's phenomenon. The mechanism may involve frank arterial occlusion or a decrease in the potential energy of blood flow to maintain blood pressure. To a lesser extent, hyperviscosity in polycythemia vera and Waldenstrom macroglobulinemia have been linked to Raynaud's phenomenon [19–25]. There is little evidence to establish hyperviscosity as a contributing factor to Raynaud's phenomenon in patients without underlying blood dyscrasias.

Neurotransmitters, hormones, and other substances released or metabolized by the endothelium, platelets, and leukocytes affect the tone of the vascular smooth muscle and therefore contribute to digital vasoconstriction, betraying their potential role in Raynaud vasospasm [3]. Serotonin, thromboxane A2, and angiotensin II have been investigated in the treatment of Raynaud's phenomenon with varying levels of support.

Other endogenous vasoactive substances and chemical markers point the way to future investigations, such as von Willebrand's factor as a marker for endothelial damage, increased polymorphonuclear leukocyte and malondialdehyde activity as a markers for increased free radical release and activity, and endothelin-1 [3].

SECONDARY CAUSES OF RAYNAUD'S PHENOMENON

Most patients encountered in the office setting have primary Raynaud's phenomenon. A small number of individuals develop these symptoms associated with other disease processes. A meta-analysis of outcomes in patients with primary Raynaud's phenomenon revealed that only 12.6% of the 639 cases reviewed developed a secondary disorder. The mean time to progress to a secondary disorder was 10.4 years after the onset of Raynaud's phenomenon [26]. In general, patients who acquire secondary disease tend to exhibit Raynaud's phenomenon later in life and have a more severe disease process. Secondary pathology includes connective tissue disorders, arterial occlusive diseases, thoracic outlet syndrome, neurologic disorders, and blood dyscrasias. Other common causes are occupational exposure to specific chemicals or consistent vibratory trauma.

Various connective tissue disorders have been associated with Raynaud's phenomenon, including scleroderma, systemic lupus erythematosus, dermatomyositis, polymyositis, mixed connective tissue disorders, and rheumatoid arthritis. Raynaud's phenomenon is more prevalent in patients with scleroderma; it is reported to occur in 80% to 90% of patient with this illness. In addition, Raynaud symptomatology is the presenting feature in 33% of patients who eventually are diagnosed as having scleroderma [3]. Patients who progress to these other rheumatologic disorders often possess deformed and enlarged capillaries noted in the nail folds. No specific test exists for predicting which patient will eventually develop a specific connective tissue disorder. A strong suspicion for a particular ailment and appropriate testing is often required to make the connection.

Diseases that occlude the arteries, such as atherosclerosis and thromboangiitis obliterans, have been identified with Raynaud's phenomenon. Patients with these illnesses possess other physical findings that point to the etiology. In addition, thoracic outlet syndrome has been associated with Raynaud's phenomenon. This condition causes compression of the nerves as they travel through the neck, which may lead to abnormalities in the vessels of the hands. Neurologic disorders including stroke, disc disease, reflex sympathetic dystrophy, and carpal tunnel syndrome have been implicated as causes of secondary Raynaud's phenomenon. Hypothyroidism has caused Raynaud's phenomenon with abatement of symptoms with thyroid replacement therapy. On rare occasions, patients with Raynaud's phenomenon suffer from cold agglutinin disease, cryoglobulinemia, or pulmonary hypertension.

Trauma to the vasculature from constant vibration causes Raynaud's phenomenon in a small number of people. Occupations involved include piano player, typist, lumbar jacks, chain saw users, and anyone who repetitively taps the fingers. It is believed that motion and percussive trauma cause endothelial damage and dysregulation, leading to vasospasm and characteristic changes in the vessel. Several drugs, including interferon, antineoplastic drugs, bromocriptine, sulphasalazine, cocaine, and tegafur, have been shown to increase a patient's propensity to develop Raynaud's phenomenon.

DIAGNOSIS OF RAYNAUD PHENOMENON

Raynaud's phenomenon is classified as the primary, idiopathic type or the secondary form that is associated with underlying pathology. The diagnosis of primary Raynaud's phenomenon is based on meeting the six criteria outlined by Allen and Brown [27] (Box 1). These criteria are based on observational studies at the Mayo Clinic, which were later reviewed by Gifford and Hines [4] (grade of recommendation: A).

The last two criteria highlight the importance of excluding connective tissue diseases, vascular pathology, and hematologic conditions. To fulfill these latter criteria or to establish a secondary diagnosis, further diagnostic testing is needed. This is important to better understand the patient's prognosis, anticipate comorbidities, and guide treatment.

Nail fold capillary microscopy can detect capillary loop deformities and avascular patches suggestive of an underlying connective tissue disorder [28,29]. Abnormal nail fold capillary pattern had a positive predictive value (PPV) of 47% and a negative predictive value (NPV) of 93% in Spencer-Green's meta-analysis (grade of recommendation: A). In this same review, presence of cutaneous lesions had a PPV of 30% and a NPV of 97% (grade of recommendation: A) [26].

Erythrocyte sedimentation rate (ESR), anti-nuclear antibody (ANA) assay, and rheumatoid factor are often performed when evaluating these patients. These screening tests, when positive, in addition to historical elements and physical examination, lead to a list of differential diagnoses that can focus the clinician's investigation into a secondary Raynaud's phenomenon. A positive ANA had a PPV of 30% and a NPV of 93% for diagnosis of connective tissue diseases (grade of recommendation: A) [26]. A Medline search failed to reveal any studies that quantify the benefit of obtaining a rheumatoid factor and an ESR for the evaluation of patients with Raynaud's phenomenon. Elevation of the ESR or a positive rheumatoid factor may prompt the clinician to look for a secondary cause.

Other frequently ordered tests for the evaluation of these patients include the identification of cryoglobulins, cold agglutinins, or predominant monoclonal bands on serum protein electrophoresis. An evaluation of the significance of low levels of cold agglutinins and cryoglobulins in patients with isolated Raynaud's phenomenon was of no diagnostic value [30] (grade of recommendation: A). A Medline search revealed no studies on the diagnostic benefit of evaluation for the presence of monoclonal bands.

Box 1. Criteria for the Diagnosis of Primary Raynaud's phenomenon

- Intermittent attacks of ischemic discoloration of the extremities
- A bilateral distribution
- Limited trophic changes to the skin without gross gangrene
- Duration of symptoms › 2 years
- Absence of organic arterial occlusion
- Absence of any symptoms or signs of systemic disease that might account for the occurrence of the phenomenon

Digital hemodynamic measurements of digital blood pressure, blood flow, and pulse volume recordings can be obtained through a variety of methods, but noninvasive vascular studies have limited diagnostic utility in differentiating primary from secondary Raynaud's phenomenon and have limited predictive value in gauging severity [3].

Although angiography is rarely indicated, it may be used to plan revascularization procedures in patients with persistent digital ischemia secondary to arterio-occlusive disorders. x-Rays of the cervical spine may be used in suspected thoracic outlet syndrome to rule out a cervical rib [3]. Table 1 lists screening tests for secondary Raynaud's phenomenon.

TREATMENT

The treatment of Raynaud's phenomenon varies depending on the type, severity, and frequency of the problem. In all cases, patients should understand that no regimen eliminates the condition but that the severity of the problem can be reduced. Treatment modalities can be divided into three categories: conservative measures, pharmacologic aids, and surgical interventions.

TABLE 1.
Screening Tests for Secondary Raynaud's Phenomenon

	Comments	Grade of Recommendation
Connective Tissue Disorders		
Antinuclear antibody	Screen and predict progression to CTDs	A
Erythrocyte sedimentation rate	Screen for CTDs	D
Rheumatoid factor	Screen for CTDs	D
Blood dyscrasias		
Cryoglobulins	No diagnostic value	Not recommended
Cold agglutinin	No diagnostic value	Not recommended
Protein electrophoresis	Identify monoclonal gammopathies	D
Miscellaneous		
Nail fold microscopy	Screen and predict progression to CTDs	A
Digital blood pressure, blood flow, and pulse volume recordings	Not recommended to differentiate primary from secondary disease	Not recommended
Angiography	Plan revascularization procedures	D
Cervical spine and chest x-ray	Evaluate for thoracic outlet syndrome if suspected	D

Abbreviation: CTD, connective tissue disease.

Conservative Measures

In mild cases, the affected individual should avoid exposure to the cold and ingestion of agents that promote changes in the blood vessels of the extremities. Benign cases can benefit from the use of warm clothing, including gloves and insulated boots. Head and body covering prevents reflex vasoconstriction of the extremities. Often, patients with these symptoms are told that tobacco use can exacerbate symptoms; however, several studies suggest that neither nicotine use nor alcohol consumption has a significant association with Raynaud's phenomenon. Stress has also been implicated as a provoking factor. Behavioral biofeedback may be helpful in controlling symptoms in some individuals (grade of recommendation: D) A skin temperature biofeedback study by Guglielmi et al [31] showed that patients reported relief of symptoms, but there was no difference in clinical measures used to assess symptomatic reprieve. Middaugh's study [32] on biofeedback techniques for patients with Raynaud's phenomenon was also inconclusive. This group determined that the effectiveness of biofeedback is related to coping skills, anxiety, gender, and clinic site. Acupuncture has more potential as a treatment modality (grade of recommendation: A). In a German trial, 33 patients were evaluated for reduction of symptoms using acupuncture. The 17 treatment patients experienced a 63% reduction in attacks as compared with a control group ($n = 16$), who experienced a 27% reduction in number of attacks [33]. Fish oil dietary supplements have also been evaluated for the management of this condition and show promise (grade of recommendation: B). These supplements improved tolerance to cold and delayed the onset of vasospasm in patients with primary Raynaud's phenomenon (Table 2) [34].

Pharmacologic Agents

Dihydropyridine types of calcium-channel blockers, such as nifedipine, have the most evidence of benefit and are recommended as first-line

TABLE 2.
Treatment Recommendations: Conservative Measures

Therapy	Comments	Grade of Recommendation
Warm clothing	Only one supporting study	D
Smoking cessation	No association with disease	
Decrease alcohol consumption	No association with disease	
Biofeedback	Improves symptom control, inconclusive	D
Acupuncture	Reduces symptoms	A
Fish oil dietary supplements	Improves tolerance to cold and delays vasospasm	B

TABLE 3.
Treatment Recommendations: Pharmacologic Interventions

Therapy	Comments	Grade of Recommendation
Calcium-channel blockers		
Nifedipine	First-line therapy; reduces symptoms and attack frequency	A
Felodipine, amlodipine, isradipine	Equally effective as nifedipine; reduces symptoms and attack frequency	A
Diltiazem, verapamil	Several studies show no benefit	Not recommended
ACE inhibitors		
Captopril	Inconclusive studies	Not recommended
Angiotensin II receptor blocker		
Losartan	Improves clinical symptoms	A
Sympathetic nervous system blockers		
Reserpine	Improves disease and ulcer healing; side effects limit long term use	A
Guanethidine, prazosin	Improves disease and ulcer healing; side effects limit long-term use	A
Phenoxybenzamine, tolazoline	May show benefit	D
Prostaglandins		
Iloprost, cisaprost, beraprost	Decrease severity and frequency of symptoms; promotes ulcer healing; inconclusive; not recommended in clinical practice	D
Serotonin antagonist		
Ketanserin	Helpful adjunctive agent, conflicting data	D
Thromboxane A2 inhibitor		
Dazoxiben	Not recommended, conflicting data	Not recommended
Vasopressin V1a	Improved symptoms to cold stimulus, inconclusive	D
Fluoxetine	Improved response to cold stimulus, inconclusive	D
Calcitonin gene-related peptide	Marginal benefit over placebo	D
Triiodothyroxine	Subjective improvement, no statistical significance, tachycardia/palpitations common	D
Cilostazol	Improved vessel diameter and response to cold; further study needed	D

TABLE 3 (*continued*).		
Therapy	**Comments**	**Grade of Recommendation**
Topically applied nitric oxide-generating systems	Increase microcirculatory flow; further study needed	D
Topical glyceryl trinitrate	Increase microcirculatory flow in secondary Raynaud's phenomenon	D

therapy (grade of recommendation: A). Nifedipine-treated patients showed a 66% reduction in verified attacks [35]. Patients experienced less severe and fewer episodes with this medication [36]. There has been some suggestion of diminishing effectiveness over time, and 30% to 61% of patients experienced side effects [37,38]. Studies have demonstrated that felodipine, amlodipine, and isradipine are equally effective in the treatment of Raynaud's phenomenon [39,40]. A related drug, nicardipine, was ineffective [41,42]. Nondihydropyridine calcium-channel blockers, such as diltiazem and verapamil, have not been shown to be useful [43–45].

Studies have not shown ACE inhibitors to be beneficial; therefore, they cannot be recommended for the treatment of symptomatic individuals. The angiotensin-2 receptor blocker losartan has been compared with nifedipine and has shown clinical improvement in patients with Raynaud's phenomenon (grade of recommendation: A) [46,47].

Sympathetic nervous system inhibitors have been adopted for therapy in Raynaud's phenomenon because the sympathetic nervous system is responsible for the vasoconstriction associated with cold and emotion. Drugs in this category include reserpine, prazosin, guanethidine, phenoxybenzamine, and tolazoline. Reserpine has been shown to improve Raynaud's phenomenon and to promote healing of digital ulcers [9] (grade of recommendation: A). The long-term benefit has been questioned, and many patients experience side effects such as nausea, lethargy, and depression. Similar agents, such as guanethidine and prazosin, initially seemed promising, but adverse effects were common [48–50]. Other agents, such as phenbenzamine and tolazoline, have shown some benefit but have not been well studied (grade of recommendation: D).

Prostaglandins are strong vasodilators that in theory may improve the symptoms of Raynaud's phenomenon. Agents in this class include iloprost, cisaprost, and beraprost. Iloprost has been the most rigorously studied agent in this class. When given intravenously, iloprost decreased the frequency and severity of attacks and promoted healing of ulcers of the heel [51,52]. After a 5-day infusion, there is evidence of prolonged physiologic improvement of the condition with the promotion of cutaneous ulcer healing despite a known mechanism. However, patient diaries describe improvement of duration and frequency of the attacks in the treatment and control groups. Oral iloprost was not significantly superior to placebo. Side affects, such as headache, flushing, nausea, and vomiting, were common [53,54]. Although these agents have shown some usefulness in clinical trials, the evidence is inconclusive. Consequently, application in clinical practice is not recommended. Serotonin antagonists are believed to decrease vasoconstriction in patients. Ketanserin, a serotonin antagonist, has been studied to determine if it is beneficial in patients with Raynaud's phenomenon. The results have been conflicting. An assessment of three trials by Pope [55] reported slight improvement in duration of attacks, but patients suffered side effects, including fatigue, edema, dry mouth, and dizziness. The authors concluded that ketanserin treatment was not clinically superior to placebo. In Lukac's [56] study of patients with systemic sclerosis, five of eight patients showed improvement. In a study by Coffman [57] of 222 patients from 10 countries, 34% of patients reported a reduction in frequency of episodes as compared with an 18% reduction in the placebo group. There was no difference in the severity of attacks [58]. Despite conflicting evidence, ketanserin is thought by some to be a helpful adjunctive therapy, especially in patients with underlying connective tissue disorders (level of recommendation: D).

Other agents have been studied less extensively. Vasopressin V1a showed improvement in symptoms during cold immersion without side effects [59]. Selective serotonin reuptake inhibitors, specifically fluoxetine, have proven valuable in response to cold challenge with few complications [60]. These agents may be future remedies, but further evaluation is needed. Calcitonin gene-related peptide, a potent vasodilator, has been speculated to be involved in the peripheral circulation's response to cold stimulus but has proven to be only slightly more beneficial than placebo in early studies [61]. The use of thromboxane inhibitors is under evaluation because thromboxane A2 causes platelet aggregation and vasoconstriction. Results are conflicting. There are some questions whether triiodothyronine would be beneficial [62]. When given triiodothyronine 80 µg daily, patients reported gradual improvement, but there was no statistically significant reduction in frequency, duration, or severity of the attacks. Four of six subjects experienced healing of skin ulcers. However, 6 of 18 subjects experienced palpitations and tachycardia, suggesting that a more physiologic dose be assessed. Cilostazol improved vessel diameter and had a favorable impact on vessel responsiveness to cold [63]. Topically applied nitric oxide-generating systems increased microcirculatory flow [64], and topical glyceryl trinitrate improved blood flow in those with secondary Raynaud's phenomenon as opposed to primary idiopathic disease [65]. These preparations are under investigation and are not recommended for use in the office setting (Table 3).

Surgical Treatments

Surgical intervention is rare but is used for patients with severe symptoms. The primary surgical technique is sympathetic nerve lysis.

TABLE 4.
Treatment Recommendations: Surgical Interventions

Therapy	Comments	Grade of Recommendation
Thoracic and lumbar sympathectomy	Decreased severity of symptoms and frequency of attacks; promotes ulcer healing; recurrence rates high	D
Digital sympathectomy	Decreases symptoms; shows long-term benefits; further evaluation needed	D
Peripheral artery adventitial stripping	Decreases symptoms; long-term benefits under investigation	D
Laser therapy	Only one study. Treatment shows promise; further evaluation needed	D

Sympathic innervation arises from T1 to T10 for the upper extremities and T10 to L2 for the lower extremities. Thoracic sympathectomy has been shown to decrease severity of attacks and promote healing of associated ulcers, but the rate of symptom recurrence is high [66]. Lumbar sympathectomy also decreases the symptoms but has a more durable outcome [67]. Digital sympathectomy and adventitial stripping of peripheral arteries have shown favorable response, but long-term outcomes are still under investigation (grade of recommendation: D) [68–70]. More recently, low-level laser therapy laser therapy has shown promise for patients with primary and secondary Raynaud's phenomenon. It is a less invasive procedure, but further evaluation of this course of action is required (Table 4) [71].

Key Points

- The average age of onset of Raynaud's Phenomenon is 31 years of age and it affects women 3 to 5 times more than men.
- Raynaud's Phenomenon is classified as either primary, idiopathic or secondary, which is associated with a secondary disease process. Most patients seen in the office setting will have primary.
- Because symptoms of Raynaud's phenomenon are intermittent the diagnosis must be made by history.
- Abnormal nail fold capillary deformity on physical exam suggests underlying pathology.
- Calcium channel blockers are considered first line of therapy in reducing symptoms and frequency of attacks.
- Surgical intervention is rare but used in patients with severe disease such as those patients with ulcers due to vasospasm.

References

[1] Coffman JD. Raynaud's phenomenon. New York: Oxford University Press; 1989.

[2] Raynaud M. L'asphyxie locale et de la Gangrene symmetrique des extremities. London: New Sydenham Society; 1862.

[3] Creager MA, Halperin JL, Coffman JD. Raynaud's phenomenon and other vascular disorders related to temperature. In: Loscalzo J, Creager MA, Dzau VJ, editors. Vascular medicine: a textbook of vascular biology and diseases. 2nd edition. Boston: Little Brown; 1996. p. 965–98.

[4] Gifford RW Jr, Hines EA Jr. Raynaud's disease among women and girls. Circulation 1957;16:1012–21.

[5] Blain A III, Coller FA, Carver GB. Raynaud's disease: a study of criteria for prognosis. Surgery 1951;29:387–97.

[6] Hines E, Christensen N. Raynaud's disease among men. JAMA 1945;129:1–4.

[7] Maricq HR, Carpentier PH, Weinrich MC, et al. Geographic variation in the prevalence of Raynaud's phenomenon: Charleston, SC, USA, vs Tarentaise, Savoie, France J Rheumatol 1993;20:70–6.

[8] Maricq HR, Weinrich MC, Keil JE, et al. Prevalence of Raynaud phenomenon in the general population: a preliminary study by questionnaire. J Chronic Dis 1986;39:423–7.

[9] Peacock JH. Peripheral venous blood concentrations of epinephrine and norepinephrine in primary Raynaud's disease. Circ Res 1959;7:821–7.

[10] Downey JA, Frewin DB. The effect of cold on blood flow in the hand of patients with Raynaud's phenomenon. Clin Sci 1973;44:279–89.

[11] Kontos HA, Wasserman AJ. Effect of reserpine in Raynaud's phenomenon. Circulation 1969;39:259–66.

[12] Vanhoutte PM, Shepherd JT. Effect of temperature on reactivity of isolated cutaneous veins of the dog. Am J Physiol 1970;218:187–90.

[13] Rusch NJ, Shepherd JT, Vanhoutte PM. The effect of profound cooling on adrenergic neurotransmission in canine cutaneous veins. J Physiol 1981;311:57–65.

[14] Vanhoutte PM, Lorenz RR. Effect of temperature on reactivity of saphenous, mesenteric, and femoral veins of the dog. Am J Physiol 1970;218:1746–50.

[15] Janssens WJ, Vanhoutte PM. Effect of cooling on efflux of [3H]-noradrenaline in canine cutaneous veins. Br J Pharmacol 1979;66:148.

[16] Janssens WJ, Vanhoutte PM. Effect of cooling on COMT activity in canine saphenous vein homogenates determined by a micro radioenzymatic assay. Arch Int Pharmacodyn Ther 1978;236:305–6.

[17] Vanhoutte PM, Cooke JP, Lindblad LE, et al. Modulation of postjunctional alpha-adrenergic responsiveness by local changes in temperature. Clin Sci 1985;68(Suppl):121S–3S.

[18] Cooke JP, Shepherd JT, Vanhoutte PM. The effect of warming on adrenergic neurotransmission in canine cutaneous vein. Circ Res 1984;54:547–53.

[19] Marshal R, Shepherd JT, Thompson I. Vascular responses in patients with high serum titres of cold agglutinins. Clin Sci 1953;12:255.

[20] Brown G, Grifin H. Peripheral arterial disease in polycythemia vera. Arch Intern Med 1930;46:705.

[21] Imhof J, Baars H, Verloop M. Clinical haematologic aspects of macroglobulinemia. Acta Med Scand 1959;163:349–66.

[22] Jager B. Cryofibrinogenemia. N Engl J Med 1962;266:579–83.

[23] McGrath MA, Peek R, Penny R. Raynaud's disease: reduced hand blood flows with normal blood viscosity. Aust N Z J Med 1978;8:126–31.

[24] Invernizzi F, Galli M, Serino G, et al. Secondary and essential cryoglobulinemias: frequency, nosological classification, and long-term follow-up. Acta Haematol 1983;70:73–82.

[25] Hillestad LK. The peripheral circulation during exposure to cold in normals and in patients with the syndrome of high-titre cold haemagglutination: I. The vascular response to cold exposure in normal subjects. Acta Med Scand 1959;164:203–29.

[26] Spencer-Green G. Outcomes in primary Raynaud phenomenon: a meta-analysis of the frequency, rates, and predictors of transition to secondary diseases. Arch Intern Med 1998;158:595–600.

[27] Allen E, Brown G. Raynaud's disease: a critical review of minimal requisites for diagnosis. Am J Med Sci 1932;183:187–200.

[28] Thompson R, Harper F, Maize J, et al. Nailfold biopsy in scleroderma and related disorders. Arthritis Rheum 1984;27:97–103.

[29] Maricq HR, Spencer-Green G, LeRoy EC. Skin capillary abnormalities as indicators of organ involvement in scleroderma (systemic sclerosis), Raynaud's syndrome and dermatomyositis. Am J Med 1976;61:862–70.

[30] Kroger K, Billen T, Neuhaus G, et al. Relevance of low titers of cryoglobulins and cold-agglutinins in patients with isolated Raynaud phenomenon. Clin Hemorheol Micro-circ 2001;24:167–74.

[31] Guglielmi RS, Roberts AH, Patterson R. Skin temperature biofeedback for Raynaud's disease: a double-blind study. Biofeedback & Self Regulation 1982;7(1):99–120.

[32] Middaugh SJ, Haythornthwaite JA, Thompson B, et al. The Raynaud's treatment study: biofeedback protocols and acquisition of temperature biofeedback skills. Applied Psychophysiology & Biofeedback 2001;26(4):251–78.

[33] Appiah R, Hiller S, Caspary L, et al. Treatment of primary Raynaud's syndrome with traditional Chinese acupuncture. J Intern Med 1997;241:119–24.

[34] DiGiacomo RA, Kremer JM, Shah DM. Fish-oil dietary supplementation in patients with Raynaud's phenomenon: a double-blind, controlled, prospective study. Am J Med 1989;86:158–64.

[35] Anonymous. Comparison of sustained-release nifedipine and temperature biofeedback for treatment of primary Raynaud phenomenon: results from a randomized clinical trial with 1-year follow-up. Arch Intern Med 2000;160:1101–8.

[36] Sarkozi J, Bookman AA, Mahon W, et al. Nifedipine in the treatment of idiopathic Raynaud's syndrome. J Rheumatol 1986;13:331–6.

[37] Gjorup T, Hartling OJ, Kelbaek H, et al. Controlled double blind trial of nisoldipine in the treatment of idiopathic Raynaud's phenomenon. Eur J Clin Pharmacol 1986;31: 387–9.

[38] Corbin DO, Wood DA, Macintyre CC, et al. A randomized double blind cross-over trial of nifedipine in the treatment of primary Raynaud's phenomenon. Eur Heart J 1986;7: 165–70.

[39] Kallenberg CG, Wouda AA, Meems L, et al. Once daily felodipine in patients with primary Raynaud's phenomenon. Eur J Clin Pharmacol 1991;40:313–5.

[40] Schmidt JF, Valentin N, Nielsen SL. The clinical effect of felodipine and nifedipine in Raynaud's phenomenon. Eur J Clin Pharmacol 1989;37:191–2.

[41] Wigley FM, Wise RA, Malamet R, et al. Nicardipine in the treatment of Raynaud's phenomenon: dissociation of platelet activation from vasospasm. Arthritis Rheum 1987;30:281–6.

[42] Anonymous. Controlled multicenter double-blind trial of nicardipine in the treatment of primary Raynaud phenomenon. French Cooperative Multicenter Group for Raynaud Phenomenon, Paris, France. Am Heart J 1991;122:352–5.

[43] da Costa J, Gomes JA, Espirito Santo J, et al. Inefficacy of diltiazem in the treatment of Raynaud's phenomenon with associated connective tissue disease: a double blind placebo controlled study. J Rheumatol 1987;14:858–9.

[44] Kinney EL, Nicholas GG, Gallo J, et al. The treatment of severe Raynaud's phenomenon with verapamil. J Clin Pharmacol 1982;22:74–6.

[45] Rhedda A, McCans J, Willan AR, et al. A double blind placebo controlled crossover randomized trial of diltiazem in Raynaud's phenomenon. J Rheumatol 1985;12:724–7.

[46] Dziadzio M, Denton CP, Smith R, et al. Losartan therapy for Raynaud's phenomenon and scleroderma: clinical and biochemical findings in a fifteen-week, randomized, parallel-group, controlled trial. Arthritis Rheum 1999;42:2646–55.

[47] Pancera P, Sansone S, Secchi S, et al. The effects of thromboxane A2 inhibition (picotamide) and angiotensin II receptor blockade (losartan) in primary Raynaud's phenomenon. J Int Med 1997;242:373–6.

[48] Pope J, Fenlon D, Thompson A, et al. Prazosin for Raynaud's phenomenon in progressive systemic sclerosis. Cochrane Database Syst Rev 2000;2: CD000956.

[49] Surwit RS, Gilgor RS, Allen LM, et al. A double-blind study of prazosin in the treatment of Raynaud's phenomenon in scleroderma. Arch Dermatol 1984;120:329–31.

[50] Russell IJ, Lessard JA. Prazosin treatment of Raynaud's phenomenon: a double blind single crossover study. J Rheumatol 1985;12:94–8.

[51] Yardumian DA, Isenberg DA, Rustin M, et al. Successful treatment of Raynaud's syndrome with iloprost, a chemically stable prostacyclin analogue. Br J Rheumatol 1988;27:220–6.

[52] Pope J, Fenlon D, Thompson A, et al. Iloprost and cisaprost for Raynaud's phenomenon in progressive systemic sclerosis. Cochrane Database Syst Rev 2000;2, CD000953.

[53] Wigley FM, Korn JH, Csuka ME, et al. Oral iloprost treatment in patients with Raynaud's phenomenon secondary to systemic sclerosis: a multicenter, placebo-controlled, double-blind study. Arthritis Rheum 1998;41:670–7.

[54] Belch JJ, Capell HA, Cooke ED, et al. Oral iloprost as a treatment for Raynaud's syndrome: a double blind multicentre placebo controlled study. Ann Rheum Dis 1995;54: 197–200.

[55] Pope J, Fenlon D, Thompson A, et al. Ketanserin for Raynaud's phenomenon in progressive systemic sclerosis. Cochrane Database Syst Rev 2000;2: CD000954.

[56] Lukac J, Rovensky J, Tauchmannova H, et al. Effect of ketanserin on Raynaud's phenomenon in progressive systemic sclerosis: a double-blind trial. Drugs Exp Clin Res 1985;11:659–63.

[57] Coffman JD, Clement DL, Creager MA, et al. International study of ketanserin in Raynaud's phenomenon. Am J Med 1989;87:264–8.

[58] Roald OK, Seem E. Treatment of Raynaud's phenomenon with ketanserin in patients with connective tissue disorders. Br Med J (Clin Res Ed) 1984;289:577–9.

[59] Hayoz D, Bizzini G, Noel B, et al. Effect of SR 49059, a V1a vasopressin receptor antagonist, in Raynaud's phenomenon. Rheumatology 2000;39:1132–8.

[60] Coleiro B, Marshall SE, Denton CP, et al. Treatment of Raynaud's phenomenon with the selective serotonin reuptake inhibitor fluoxetine. Rheumatology 2001;40:1038–43.

[61] Bunker CB, Reavley C, O'Shaughnessy DJ, et al. Calcitonin gene-related peptide in treatment of severe peripheral vascular insufficiency in Raynaud's phenomenon. Lancet 1993;342:80–3.

[62] Dessein PH, Morrison RC, Lamparelli RD, et al. Triiodothyronine treatment for Raynaud's phenomenon: a controlled trial. J Rheumatol 1990;17:1025–8.

[63] Rajagopalan S, Pfenninger D, Somers E, et al. Effects of cilostazol in patients with Raynaud's syndrome. Am J Cardiol 2003;92:1310–5.

[64] Tucker AT, Pearson RM, Cooke ED, et al. Effect of nitric-oxide-generating system on microcirculatory blood flow in skin of patients with severe Raynaud's syndrome: a randomised trial. Lancet 1999;354:1670–5.

[65] Coppock JS, Hardman JM, Bacon PA, et al. Objective relief of vasospasm by glyceryl trinitrate in secondary Raynaud's phenomenon. Postgrad Med J 1986;62:15–8.

[66] Matsumoto Y, Ueyama T, Endo M, et al. Endoscopic thoracic sympathectomy for Raynaud's phenomenon. J Vasc Surg 2002;36:57–61.

[67] Janoff KA, Phinney ES, Porter JM. Lumbar sympathectomy for lower extremity vasospasm. Am J Surg 1985;150:147–52.

[68] Balogh B, Mayer W, Vesely M, et al. Adventitial stripping of the radial and ulnar arteries in Raynaud's disease. J Hand Surg 2002;27:1073–80.

[69] Tomaino MM, Goitz RJ, Medsger TA. Surgery for ischemic pain and Raynaud's' phenomenon in scleroderma: a description of treatment protocol and evaluation of results. Microsurgery 2001;21:75–9.

[70] Yee AM, Hotchkiss RN, Paget SA. Adventitial stripping: a digit saving procedure in refractory Raynaud's phenomenon. J Rheumatol 1998;25:269–76.

[71] al-Awami M, Schillinger M, Maca T, et al. Low level laser therapy for treatment of primary and secondary Raynaud's phenomenon. Vasa 2004;33:25–9.

Address reprint requests to

Dyanne Westerberg
Christiana Care Health Services
1401 Foulk Road, Wilmington, DE 19803

e-mail: Dwesterberg@christianacare.org

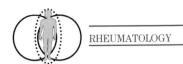

RHEUMATOLOGY   1522–5720/05 $15.00 + .00

A PRIMARY CARE APPROACH TO THE USE AND INTERPRETATION OF COMMON RHEUMATOLOGIC TESTS

Brooke E. Salzman, MD, Janice E. Nevin, MD, MPH, and James H. Newman, MD, FACP

The results of common rheumatologic laboratory tests play an important part in the diagnosis and management of rheumatic diseases. Rheumatologic test results can often be ambiguous and can sometimes be misleading, particularly in primary care settings. Because the diagnosis of most rheumatic conditions depends on information derived from sources other than serum tests, these laboratory values are usually supportive rather than diagnostic [1]. Few serum test results are pathognomonic for a specific rheumatic disease and alone are insufficient to determine a diagnosis [2]. Test results should be interpreted in a clinical context, which includes information derived from the history and physical examination, basic laboratory tests, radiographic and other imaging studies, and synovial fluid analysis. Serum rheumatologic tests are most useful for confirming a clinically suspected diagnosis. Because there is a high incidence of false-positive results in the general population, these tests have little clinical utility when there is a low pretest probability. Furthermore, the predictive value of serum rheumatologic tests is limited when performed in settings in which the prevalence of rheumatic conditions is low.

Studies suggest that primary care physicians overuse common rheumatologic tests [3]. The practice of routinely ordering a battery of rheumatologic laboratory tests to "rule out" rheumatologic disease is not uncommon [1]. This approach rarely leads to a definitive diagnosis and

From the Department of Family Medicine, Thomas Jefferson University Hospital, Philadelphia, Pennsylvania (BES); The Department of Family and Community Medicine, Christiana Care Health System, Wilmington, Delaware (JEN); Jefferson Medical College, Philadelphia, Pennsylvania (JHN); and the Section of Rheumatology, Christiana Care Health System, Wilmington, Delaware (JHN) usually increases diagnostic confusion. The significant proportion of false-positive test results, especially among elderly patients, contributes to this confusion. The misapplication of rheumatologic tests can lead to mis-diagnoses, unnecessary work-ups, needless referrals and treatments, and increased health care costs. The overuse of such tests reduces their pre-dictive value in the primary care setting.

Patients with musculoskeletal complaints and constitutional symp-toms (eg, fatigue) are commonly evaluated by primary care physicians. The vast majority of these patients do not have a rheumatologic disease [4]. The use of rheumatologic tests by primary care doctors may be improved by increasing understanding regarding the indications for and value of such tests. Recognizing the limitations of rheumatologic tests may improve their utility by encouraging more selective testing and more cautious inter-pretation of test results [5]. This article describes the characteristics of commonly ordered rheumatologic tests and reviews examples of their application in a primary care setting.

DEFINITIONS OF STATISTICAL TERMS

To fully understand the clinical utility of a test, it is important to have an understanding of fundamental test characteristics and their application in a clinical setting. Performance attributes of a test include sensitivity, specificity, positive predictive values (PPVs), and negative predictive values (NPVs). Sensitivity refers to the percentage of patients with the disease who have a positive test result. For example, about 80% of patients with rheumatoid arthritis (RA) are positive for rheumatoid factor (RF). Conversely, 20% of patients with RA have a negative test result for RF (false-negative result). Specificity refers to the percentage of patients without the disease who have a negative test result. Patients without the disease with a positive test result have a false-positive result.

Sensitivity and specificity can be affected by the clinical setting in which the test is performed. For example, only about one third of RA patients develop RF in the first 3 months of illness [4]. Therefore, for the primary care physician who is likely to evaluate a patient with RA early in the course of the disease, the sensitivity of RF for RA may be lower than for a rheumatologist, who is likely to evaluate the patient at a later stage of the condition [4]. In addition, sensitivity and specificity can be affected by characteristics of patient populations. For instance, the specificity of antinuclear antibody (ANA) tests can be lower among inpatients than among outpatients because hospitalized patients are more likely to have other conditions associated with a false-positive ANA test [4]. The sen-sitivity and specificity of a given test can change depending on the defi-nition of the normal and abnormal range [4]. A wider normal range may increase the specificity of a test by reducing the number of false-positive results but can reduce its sensitivity. Conversely, a wider abnormal range may increase a test's sensitivity but may decrease its specificity. Choosing the value that distinguishes normal from abnormal involves balancing the importance of a test's sensitivity and specificity.

Although sensitivity and specificity are informative measures of test performance, they cannot inform clinicians of the probability that an individual patient has the disease in question because these test characteristics are determined from patients who are known to have or not have the disease. In practice, clinicians may not know a patient's true disease state. Therefore, the test feature of relevance to practicing clinicians is a test's ability to estimate the probability that a patient has the disease in question. The PPV is the probability that the patient has the disease given a positive test result. The NPV is the probability that the patient does not have the disease given a negative result.

The predictive value of a test is influenced by the clinical context in which it is applied. The predictive value may be calculated using Bayes' theorem, which relies upon the test sensitivity, test specificity, and the patient's pretest probability. A patient's pretest probability is estimated by using elements of the history, physical examination and other diagnostic data, and the prevalence of the disease in the population. The pretest probability has significant bearing on the ability of a test to predict the probability of disease. Even if a test has excellent sensitivity and specificity, a test used in a patient with a low pretest probability may have poor predictive value [6].

ISSUES IN LABORATORY TESTS IN RHEUMATOLOGY

Titers

There are a number of special features intrinsic to rheumatologic laboratory tests that should be considered when interpreting their meaning. First, many rheumatologic tests, such as RF and ANA tests, are reported in a quantitative fashion using a serum dilution titer. The reported titer represents the highest dilution of serum that yields detectable agglutination. The incidence of a positive result in a population depends on the assay system used and the titer chosen to separate positive and negative responses [7]. The titer selected to distinguish between normal and abnormal should be based on the disease prevalence in the patient's local population. Often, the cutoff dilution is intended to exclude 95% of the normal population while maintaining a test's sensitivity for disease. Each laboratory must determine the level it considers positive, and this level may vary significantly between labs. In general, the higher the titer is, the lower the false-positive rate. The converse is also true: the lower the titer is, the higher the false-positive rate of the test.

Guidelines constructed by the American College of Rheumatology Ad Hoc Committee on Immunologic Testing recommend that test results like ANA should not only be reported as "positive" or "negative" but should also give an account of the highest titer for which antibody is detected. The committee submits that laboratory reports should also disclose the percentage of patients without any ANA-associated disease who have similar titers [8].

Crossreactivity

Another important issue in the ordering of rheumatologic tests is the high rate of crossreactivity [4]. Several different rheumatic conditions that share symptomatology and presentation may cause positive test results for various distinct diseases. For example, RA and systemic lupus erythematosus (SLE) may present with symmetric polyarthritis. ANA testing ordered to evaluate for SLE will be positive in 30% or more of patients with RA [4]. Thus, such cross-reactivity may lower the PPV of ANA testing for the diagnosis of SLE.

Interlaboratory Variability

Interlaboratory variability in rheumatologic testing and in measurement error contributes to the difficult task of interpreting lab results [1,4,7]. In one study, two university immunology laboratories differed in their classification of duplicate serum samples as normal or abnormal in 11% of cases for ANA testing, in 15% of cases for DNA binding testing, and in 27% of cases for serum complement testing [9]. Heterogeneity among test results between laboratories may be a consequence of variability in methods, substrates, reagents, visualizing equipment, and the subjective component of reading results [10]. Although there are efforts to standardize laboratory technique and minimize measurement error [2], test results need to be interpreted in consideration of individual laboratory methodology. If a laboratory value does not agree with the clinical estimation, the clinician may consider laboratory error to explain the finding [1].

Testing Bias and Generalizability

Laboratory test performance in the general population can be difficult to determine when studies evaluating such tests examine populations with dissimilar disease prevalence or varying levels of suspected disease [1,10]. For instance, many studies investigating the properties of rheumatologic tests include a selected group of patients who have been referred to a rheumatologist and who may have a specific constellation of symptoms [10]. Therefore, applying data regarding the value of these tests to the general population or to a primary care setting can be problematic.

Rheumatoid Factor

RF is one of the most commonly ordered tests in the evaluation of patients with musculoskeletal complaints. Most RFs are IgM autoantibodies, which bind to the Fc portion of IgG immunoglobulins. Although the diagnosis of RA cannot be made on the basis of RF testing alone, a positive RF is included among the American College of Rheumatology criteria for the diagnosis of RA [11]. The sensitivity of RF is about 80% in patients with RA, although studies have reported rates ranging from 30% to 90% [12]. Some authors suggest that 80% may be an overestimate due to selection bias because studies may have intended to include indisputable and possibly more severe cases of RA [5]. The specificity of RF for RA ranges from 80% to 98%, depending on the study [12] and the age and health of the population studied [6]. The titer of RF also differs among various ethnic groups [13]. Patients with elderly-onset RA and female patients are more often seronegative [5].

A false-positive RF is found in a number of other rheumatic and nonrheumatic conditions (Box 1). Several of these conditions may present

---

Box 1. Conditions Commonly Associated with a Positive Rheumatoid Factor

Rheumatic diseases (prevalence)
- Rheumatoid arthritis (50% to 90%)
- Systemic lupus erythematosus (15% to 35%)
- Sjögren's syndrome (75% to 95%)
- Systemic sclerosis (20% to 30%)
- Polymyositis/dermatomyositis (5% to 10%)
- Cryoglobulinemia (40% to 100%)
- Mixed connective tissue disease (50% to 60%)

Nonrheumatic conditions
- Aging (> 70 years) (10% to 25%)
- Infections
  Bacterial endocarditis (25% to 50%)
  Hepatitis (15% to 40%)
  Tuberculosis (8%)
  Syphilis (up to 13%)
  Parasitic diseases (20% to 90%)
  Leprosy (5% to 58%)
  Viral infections (15% to 65%; including mumps, rubella, influenza, HIV, mononucleosis, and many others)
- Pulmonary diseases
  Sarcoidosis (3% to 33%)
  Interstitial pulmonary fibrosis (10% to 50%)
  Silicosis (30% to 50%)
  Asbestosis (30%)
- Miscellaneous diseases
  Primary biliary cirrhosis (45% to 70%)
  Malignancy (5% to 25%)

Adapted from Shmerling R, Delbanco T. The rheumatoid factor: an analysis of clinical utility. Am J Med 1991;91:528–34; with permission.

with similar musculoskeletal complaints, thereby adding to the diagnostic confusion. However, RF titers in patients with nonrheumatic conditions tend to be lower than in RA [13]. Unexplained positive RF titers may suggest underlying hepatitis C, multiple myeloma, lymphoma, or sarcoidosis. RF also occurs in normal individuals. The prevalence of RF in the normal population is at least 1%, although this figure may rise with age, reaching 10% to 25% in healthy elderly patients [4,5,14]. Because the prevalence of RA ranges from 0.5% to 3%, at least as many individuals who have a positive RF do not have RA as have the disease [1,5].

The presence of RF has often been misinterpreted as being diagnostic for RA. The clinician's estimated pretest probability that a patient has RA greatly affects the ability of RFs to aid in diagnosis. For instance, if a clinician were to use RF as a screening test, assuming a 1% pretest probability based on the prevalence of RA in the general population, a test sensitivity of 80%, and a specificity of 95%, the PPV of the RF is only 16%. This means that there is only a 16% chance that a patient with a positive RF has RA (Table 1). On the other hand, if a clinician estimated that the pretest probability of a patient having RA was 25%, a positive RF would increase the probability of RA to 84% (Table 1). Therefore, the selection of patients with a sufficient pretest probability improves the test's utility. RF testing is most useful when there is a moderate level of suspicion for RA.

When the clinical suspicion for RA is high, RF testing is less helpful because 20% of patients with RA are seronegative [6]. False-negative rates are even more common early in the course of RA. RF is detectable in only 33% of patients who develop RF during the first 3 months of disease and in only 60% of patients who develop RF during the first 6 months [1]. This may be particularly relevant in a primary care setting, where patients are evaluated earlier in the course of disease. Therefore, if there is a high probability that a patient has RA, that patient has a reasonable chance of having

TABLE 1.
Predictive Value of Rheumatic Factor for Rheumatoid Arthritis[a]

Pretest Probability	Post-test Probability, RF(+)	Post-test Probability, RF(-)
1%[b]	16%	0.2%
15%	74%	4%
25%	84%	7%
50%	94%	17%
75%	98%	39%
90%	99%	65%

Abbreviation: RF, rheumatic factor.
From Shmerling R, Delbanco T. The rheumatoid factor: an analysis of clinical utility. Am J Med 1991;91:528–34; with permission.
[a] Assuming that the sensitivity of RF is 80% and the specificity is 95%.
[b] Based on the estimated prevalence of RA in the US of 0.5% to 3%.

RA even with a negative RF (Table 1). In these cases, RF testing may lead a physician away from the diagnosis of RA, which is regrettable as more evidence demonstrates the importance of treating RA early, before end-organ damage.

In patients with RA, the RF titer generally correlates with severe articular disease and extra-articular manifestations, although this relationship is variable. RF testing may have prognostic value in these patients [6,15]. However, RF titers are not helpful in following disease progression. Once a patient has a positive RF test, repeating the test is of no value [6].

Few studies have addressed the utility of using RF testing in diseases other than RA. RF is often positive in Sjögren's syndrome and cryoglobulinemia and can be useful when these conditions are suspected. Because the presence of cryoglobulins can be difficult to confirm, RF testing can sometimes be used as a surrogate when cryoglobulinemia is suspected. It has been suggested that the disappearance of the RF in a patient with Sjögren's syndrome may indicate the onset of lymphoma [6]. In addition, RF is often ordered in the evaluation of fever of unknown origin (FUO). The utility of RF testing in FUO has been questioned in consideration of the infrequency of prolonged fever in RA and the low yield of RF testing in such cases [5].

Antinuclear Antibody

ANA testing is the most commonly performed autoantibody test in clinical laboratories [16]. It is usually ordered to evaluate for the presence of SLE or other connective tissue diseases (CTDs). The ANA test detects antibodies that bind to various nuclear and cytoplasmic antigens. Most ANA testing uses an indirect immunofluorescence technique for the initial screening test, although ELISA tests are available. Although substrates can differ between labs, most labs use HEp-2 cells over traditional rodent tissues because of their improved sensitivity.

When an ANA test is positive (titers $\geq 1:160$), the nuclear staining pattern is frequently reported. This pattern reflects the intracellular target of the nuclear antibody and may convey clinically useful information. Nuclear patterns include homogenous/diffuse, rim/peripheral, speckled, nucleolar, and centromere. These patterns have been associated with specific CTDs; however, there is substantial overlap and variation between diseases and patterns. The homogenous and rim pattern is characteristic for SLE [16]. A speckled pattern can occur with Sjögren's syndrome and mixed CTD. A nucleolar pattern is associated with diffuse scleroderma, and a centromere pattern is specific for CREST syndrome (calcinosis cutis, Raynaud's phenomenon, esophageal dysmotility, sclerodactyly, and telangiectasias) [16].

Emphasis on nuclear staining patterns has diminished over the past several years because of their lack of specificity and the availability of more specific autoantibody tests [2,17]. Furthermore, fluorescent patterns may vary with serum dilution, which may limit their reliability and reproducibility [18,19]. In addition, traditional nuclear staining patterns may differ with ANA testing using newer HEp-2 cell substrates [2].

The nuclear pattern and titer of ANA tests do not necessarily reflect disease activity. Therefore, the ANA test is most useful for diagnostic purposes and has no utility for monitoring patients. Serial ANA testing has no known value in patients with a positive ANA. Other laboratory tests (eg, complement, anti-double-stranded DNA antibodies, and erythrocyte sedimentation rate [ESR]) are more useful in assessing disease activity. Clinical factors, including patient symptoms and physical examination findings, and the results of routine laboratory values, including a CBC, creatinine, and urinalysis, are also much more significant in assessing disease activity.

An ANA titer is the primary laboratory test used to diagnose SLE. The ANA test is sensitive for SLE, with about 95% to 100% of patients with SLE having positive results [10]. A positive ANA is included in the updated American College of Rheumatology criteria for the diagnosis of SLE [20–22]. A positive test alone is insufficient for the diagnosis. Before the diagnosis of SLE can be established, 4 of 11 clinical and laboratory criteria must be met (Box 2). The ANA test is not specific for SLE. Reported specificities range from 49% to 90% [6,10].

ANA testing has a role in the diagnosis of other CTDs. A positive ANA test is required for the diagnosis of some rheumatic conditions, including drug-induced lupus, autoimmune hepatitis, and mixed CTD [2,10]. The ANA test can be positive in other CTDs, such as scleroderma, Sjögren's syndrome, and polymyositis/dermatomyositis, in varying degrees (Table 2). In these conditions, a positive ANA test can support the diagnosis but

---

Box 2. The American College of Rheumatology Criteria for Systemic Lupus Erythematosus (abbreviated)

Malar rash—Flat or raised fixed erythema

Discoid rash—Raised patches with plugging/scaling

Photosensitivity—Photosensitive skin rash

Oral ulcers—Usually painless

Nonerosive arthritis—Involving two or more peripheral joints

Serositis—Pleural or cardiac

Renal disease—Proteinuria or cellular casts

Neurologic disorder—Seizures or psychosis in the absence of other cause

Hematologic disorder—Hemolytic anemia, leukopenia, lymphopenia, thrombocytopenia

Immunologic disorder—Anti-dsDNA, anti-Sm, antiphospholipid antibodies (anticardiolipin antibody, lupus anticoagulant, or a false-positive venereal disease reference laboratory test)

Antinuclear antibody—Abnormal titer of antinuclear antibody by immunofluorescence or an equivalent assay at any point in time in the absence of drug

Data from references 19–21.

TABLE 2.
Conditions Associated with a Positive Antinuclear Antibody (ANA Test)

Rheumatic Conditions[a]	Patients with positive ANA
Systemic lupus erthematosus	99%
Drug-induced lupus	100%
Scleroderma/systemic sclerosis	97%
Mixed connective tissue disease	93%
Polymyositis/dermatomyositis	78%
Sjögren's syndrome	96%
Rheumatoid arthritis	40%
Nonrheumatic Conditions[b]	
Normal individuals: females > males, increasing age, relatives of patients with rheumatic disease, pregnancy	
Hepatic diseases: chronic active hepatitis, primary biliary cirrhosis, alcoholic liver disease	
Pulmonary diseases: idiopathic pulmonary fibrosis, asbestosis, primary pulmonary hypertension	
Chronic infections	
Malignancies: lymphoma, leukemia, melanoma, solid tumors (ovary, breast, lung, kidney)	
Hematologic disorders: idiopathic thrombocytopenic purpura, autoimmune hemolytic anemia	
Miscellaneous: type 1 diabetes mellitus, Grave disease, multiple sclerosis, end-stage renal failure, after organ transplantation	

[a] *Adapted from* Peng S, Craft J. Antinuclear antibodies. In: Ruddy S, Harris E, Sledge C, editors. Kelly's textbook of rheumatology. 6th edition. Philadelphia: Saunders; 2001: p. 161–73; with permission.
[b] *Adapted from* Pincus T. Laboratory tests in rheumatic disorders. In: Klippel J, Dieppe P, editors. Rheumatology. 2nd edition. Philadelphia: Mosby; 1998. p. 10.5.

is not required [2]. An ANA test is positive in approximately 40% to 50% of patients with antiphospholipid antibody syndrome, and its presence may increase the likelihood that the syndrome is secondary to SLE, but a positive ANA test is not necessary for the diagnosis [2,7]. Although a positive ANA test is not uncommon in patients with RA, its presence has no diagnostic significance in RA and is not useful in patients suspected of having RA [10].

Although the ANA test is not useful for establishing the diagnosis of Raynaud's phenomenon or juvenile chronic arthritis (JCA), the presence of a positive ANA test with these conditions may provide information concerning prognosis. A positive ANA test result in a patient with Raynaud's phenomenon increases the likelihood of the development of a systemic rheumatic disease from around 19% to 30%, whereas a negative ANA test result decreases the likelihood to approximately 7% [2]. Thus, a negative ANA test in this case may be reassuring. The presence of a positive ANA test result in children with JCA may predict the development of uveitis and should prompt screening [2].

Because of the high sensitivity of the ANA test for SLE, almost all patients with SLE have a positive ANA test. However, due to the low prevalence of SLE in the general population (40–50 cases per 100,000), most patients with a positive ANA test do not have SLE [2]. ANA tests can be positive in many nonrheumatic conditions and among normal individuals, particularly in women and in elderly persons (Table 2). Positive ANA tests have been noted during pregnancy and in patients with silicone gel implants [6]. In addition, up to 30% of relatives of patients with CTD may have high titers of ANA without having manifestations of disease [10,19]. Studies have shown that nearly 32% of normal individuals have a positive ANA at a 1:40 serum dilution, 13% have a positive ANA at a 1:80 serum dilution, 5% have a positive ANA at a 1:160 serum dilution, and 3% have a positive ANA at a 1:320 serum dilution [7,10,23]. Although the American College of Rheumatology criteria refer to an "abnormal" ANA titer, there is no set titer value that can distinguish between those with and without SLE. Titers >1:320 are more likely to represent true-positive results [2]. Each laboratory must determine the level that it considers positive, and this level may vary significantly among laboratories depending on various methodologic variables [16]. In most laboratories, the level of a positive ANA titer is 1:40 to 1:80. In laboratories where HEp-2 cells are used as substrates to perform an ANA test, titers of 1:80 or higher are considered positive [2]. Although each laboratory should establish its own reference intervals, guidelines suggest that titers <1:40 are negative and that titers ≥1:160 are positive [24]. Titers ≥1:40 and <1:160 are weakly positive and are common in healthy individuals. Such titers need to be interpreted in their clinical context. In the absence of specific symptoms suggesting CTD, further diagnostic study is not advised [24,25]. Although using higher cutoffs to define a positive ANA titer may improve the specificity of the test for the diagnosis of SLE, this practice would decrease its diagnostic sensitivity.

False-positive results of ANA testing constitute one of the most common reasons for rheumatology consultations [1]. If one considers that positive ANAs appear in at least 5% of the normal population and that SLE occurs in only about 40 to 50 cases per 100,000 persons, the likelihood of a positive ANA result indicating the presence of SLE is low. Studies estimate that the PPV of the ANA test in the general population is only 11% [9]. This means that a positive ANA is indicative of rheumatic disease in only 11% of patients and may have no clinical significance in nearly 90% of patients. An ANA test should be ordered if the clinician feels there is a reasonable clinical suspicion of SLE or another CTD based on the patient's history, physical examination findings, and results of other laboratory tests or studies [2]. Because most patients with a positive ANA test do not have SLE or any other rheumatic disease, ANA testing is not recommend as a screening test to rule out rheumatic disease, particularly when the suspicion for disease is low.

A negative ANA test has a high NPV and usually indicates the absence of SLE or other CTDs. Evidence suggests that testing for specific autoantibodies after a negative ANA result or after a weakly positive ANA (<1:160) is not helpful and yields positive results in fewer than 5% of cases [25]. A proportion of patients can have a negative ANA titer early in the course of disease and eventually develop a positive ANA titer [20]. Therefore, it can be worthwhile to repeat the ANA test if the patient's clinical course develops features consistent with a CTD. In rare instances, patients with SLE can have a negative ANA test. This can occur if the substrate used in the fluorescent ANA test did not contain sufficient antigen to allow for detection of those antibodies, usually the antigen Ro/SS-A. However, with more routine use of HEp-2 cell substrates, virtually all SLE patients have a positive ANA test [2]. If the clinical picture strongly suggests CTD and if the ANA is negative, further investigation should include testing for specific assays for Ro, La, Jo-1, and phospholipids [18]. Complement studies, including testing for C3, C4, and CH50, may be indicated because complement deficiencies can cause an ANA-negative, lupus-like syndrome [26].

Because specific autoantibody tests possess diagnostic significance, a positive ANA usually warrants follow-up with specialized assays (Table 3) [40]. If SLE is suspected, further work-up may include tests for anti-dsDNA, anti-Sm, anti-U1 snRNP, anti-Ro, and anti-La antibodies [18]. If mixed CTD is suspected, the serum should be tested for anti-U1 RNP antibodies; for Sjögren's syndrome, the serum should be tested for anti-Ro and anti-La antibodies; in scleroderma, the serum should be tested for anti-Scl-70 (or topoisomerase I) and anti-centromere antibodies; and in polymyositis/dermatomyositis, the serum should be tested for anti-Jo-1 antibodies. The ordering of specific autoantibodies should be targeted to address a suspected diagnosis, rather than including a large panel of tests with uncertain significance.

INFLAMMATORY MARKERS: ERYTHROCYTE SEDIMENTATION RATE AND C-REACTIVE PROTEIN

The systemic response to tissue injury, regardless of the cause, is characterized by a cytokine-mediated alteration in the hepatic synthesis of a number of different plasma proteins, known collectively as "acute phase reactants" [27]. These proteins, which include fibrinogen, C-reactive protein (CRP), serum amyloid A protein, and many others, rise in proportion to the severity of tissue injury, although the magnitude of each component varies. Because some systemic rheumatic conditions cause tissue inflammation and injury, assessment of the acute phase response can play an important part in the diagnosis and management of these diseases [27].

Laboratory tests, including erythrocyte sedimentation rate (ESR) and CRP, are commonly used to measure systemic inflammation or the acute phase response. These tests may help assess the degree of disease activity in some rheumatic conditions and monitor disease activity and response to treatment over time [28]. ESR and CRP levels may have prognostic value in conditions such as RA. Studies suggest that ESR and CRP levels are associated with long-term outcomes of RA, such as work disability [29,30]

TABLE 3.
Other Autoantibodies Detected in Patients with Connective Tissue Diseases

Autoantibody	Disease (percentage)	Comments
Anti-dsDNA	Active SLE (60–70) Inactive SLE (20)	Specific but less sensitive for SLE; correlates with lupus nephritis and disease activity. Tests for single-stranded DNA are nonspecific and should not be ordered.
Anti-histone	Absent in drug-induced lupus Drug-induced lupus (95) Idiopathic SLE (>50)	Sensitive but nonspecific for drug-induced lupus
Anti-U1 snRNP	SLE (35–40), mixed connective tissue disease (100)	Nonspecific; part of the criteria for MCTD; associated with milder disease and less nephritis
Anti-Sm	SLE (20–30)	Highly specific but not sensitive for SLE
Anti-Ro (anti-SS-A)	Sjögren's syndrome (60–75), SLE (40)	Associated with "ANA-negative" SLE, cutaneous involvement, congenital heart block in babies of mothers with this antibody [17]
Anti-La (anti-SS-B)	Sjögren's syndrome (50), SLE (10–15)	Usually occurs with anti-Ro; associated with late-onset SLE, secondary Sjögren's, neonatal lupus syndrome [6]
Anti-ribosome	SLE (10–20)	Highly specific but not sensitive for SLE; correlated with neuropsychiatric SLE [6]

Anti-centromere	Scleroderma (22–36) [6] CREST variant (80–90) PSS (25)	Associated with limited scleroderma (CREST) and Raynaud's phenomenon
Anti-topoisomerase I (Anti-ScL-70)	Scleroderma (22–40) [6] PSS (30)	Specific but not sensitive for scleroderma; correlated with progressive systemic sclerosis
Anti-Jo 1	Polymyositis and dermatomyositis (20–30)	Highly specific but not sensitive for polymyositis/dermatomyositis; associated with pulmonary fibrosis and Raynaud's phenomenon [6]
Antiphospholipid ACA, Lupus anticoagulant	ACA: SLE (12–30) [40] Lupus anticoagulant: SLE (15–34) [40]	Associated with thrombosis, thrombocytopenia, recurrent fetal loss, livedo reticularis

Abbreviations: ACA, anticardiolipin; ANA, antinuclear antibody; MCTD, mixed connective tissue disease; PSS, progressive systemic sclerosis; SLE, systemic lupus erythematosus.

Adapted from Snow C. Laboratory testing for musculoskeletal diseases. In: Harris E, Genovese M, editors. Primary care rheumatology. Philadelphia: WB Saunders; 2000; p. 55; with permission.

and radiologic progression of RA [30,31]. These inflammatory markers could allow physicians to identify patients at greatest risk for progressive disease so they can be treated more aggressively.

Generally, ESR and CRP are nonspecific indicators of inflammation and are not useful as screening tests for rheumatic conditions [32]; nor are they helpful for differentiating various rheumatic diseases [32]. However, in addition to assessing disease activity, they can be helpful for supporting the diagnosis of some rheumatic diseases, such as temporal/giant cell arteritis, polymyalgia rheumatica (PMR), and RA.

Erythrocyte Sedimentation Rate

ESR is a simple and inexpensive laboratory test that is commonly ordered in clinical medicine [33]. Although a single ESR test is inexpensive to perform, the test is ordered so frequently that it becomes expensive in the aggregate [32]. The ESR is an indirect measure of inflammation. The test measures the distance that erythrocytes have fallen after 1 hour in a vertical column of anticoagulated blood under the influence of gravity [27]. The most accurate method of performing the ESR was introduced by Westergren in 1921 [33].

TABLE 4.
Factors that May Influence the Erythrocyte Sedimentation Rate

Increase ESR	Decrease ESR
Anemia	Red blood cell abnormalities: sickle cell disease, anisocytosis
Hypercholesterolemia	Spherocytosis: acanthocytosis, microcytosis
Female sex	Extreme leukocytosis
Pregnancy	Polycythemia
Old age	Bile salts
Technical factors: dilutional problem, tilted ESR tube, increased temperature of specimen	Technical factors: dilutional problem, inadequate mixing, clotting of blood sample, short ESR tube, vibration during test, >2 h delay in running the test, low temperature of specimen
Elevated fibrinogen level: infection, inflammation, malignancy, chronic renal failure, tissue damage (MI, CVA)	Protein abnormalities: hypofibrinogenemia, hypogammaglobulinemia, dysproteinemia with hyperviscosity
Red blood cell abnormalities: macrocytosis	High doses of adrenal steroids

Abbreviations: CVA, cerebrovascular accident; ESR, erythrocyte sedimentation rate; MI, myocardial infarction.
Adapted from Bridgen M. Clinical utility of the erythrocyte sedimentation rate. Am Fam Physician 1999;60:1443–50; with permission.

An elevated ESR is a nonspecific finding. There are many conditions and factors that influence the level of ESR (Table 4). Sedimentation of erythrocytes is facilitated by certain plasma proteins that neutralize the negative charge on the erythrocyte surface, permitting them to aggregate and fall more rapidly as a clump rather than as individual cells [32]. Fibrinogen is among the plasma proteins associated with the acute phase response that acts in this regard. The amount of fibrinogen in the blood directly correlates with the ESR. Conditions that elevate fibrinogen (eg, pregnancy, diabetes, renal failure, heart disease, CTD, or malignancy) may elevate the ESR [33]. Other proteins not associated with the acute phase response (eg, immunoglobulins) can elevate the ESR. Monoclonal or polyclonal gammopathies, including multiple myeloma, can cause an elevated ESR. Anemia and macrocytosis increase the ESR.

Normal ESR values span a wide range, with women, elderly individuals, and obese individuals tending to have higher ESR values. Many individuals 70 years of age and older may have ESRs in the range of 40 to 50 mm/h without apparent inflammation or tissue injury, which limits the utility of ESR testing in the elderly population. Researchers have developed an empirical formula to estimate the value of ESR that includes 98% of healthy individuals: For men, age in years is divided by two; for women, age in years plus 10 is divided by two [32]. As with other laboratory tests, the reference range used for the ESR should be established by the laboratory performing the test (Table 5) [41]. There are several technical factors regarding the performance of the ESR test that may produce erroneous values (Table 4).

Because an elevated ESR may occur in many different clinical settings, this finding may be irrelevant as an isolated laboratory value [33]. The cause of most ESR elevations can be revealed through a detailed history, physical examination, and collection of routine laboratory data [32,33]. Most unexplained ESR elevations are short lived and are not associated with a specific underlying process [32]. An unexplained elevated ESR returns to normal in most cases. Therefore, unexplained

TABLE 5.
Reference Ranges for the Erythrocyte Sedimentation Rate in Healthy Adults

Adults	Upper Limit of Reference Range (mm/h)
Age <50 yr	
Men	0–15
Women	0–25
Age >50 yr	
Men	0–20
Women	0–30

Data from Bottiger L, Svedberg C. Normal erythrocyte sedimentation rate and age. Br Med J 1967;2:85–7; with permission.

elevated ESR levels can be rechecked in 1 to 3 months, rather than triggering an extensive search for a cause [32].

The false-positive rate is lower for an extreme elevation of ESR, defined as > 100 mm/h. In most of these cases, the condition causing the elevated ESR is clinically apparent; no obvious cause is identified in < 2% of patients [32]. An exhaustive search for an occult malignancy in patients with ESR levels > 100 mm/h is not recommended because if cancer is present it is almost always metastatic [32]. Conversely, an ESR test is often normal in the presence of various diseases, including malignancies and rheumatic conditions. Therefore, it has limited value as a test to exclude serious conditions [32].

An elevated ESR remains an important diagnostic criterion for two rheumatic conditions: PMR and temporal/giant cell arteritis [33]. Most patients with these conditions have an elevated ESR [32]. Occasionally, patients may present with a normal value. If there is good clinical evidence for these conditions, a normal ESR should not preclude the diagnosis [32].

An ESR of at least 40 mm/h has been included in the diagnostic criteria of PMR [34,35]. However, some studies have reported that the percentage of patients with PMR who have an ESR lower than 40 mm/h is about 20% [34,35]. Patients with PMR with low ESRs were more likely to be men, were generally younger, had fewer systemic manifestations, and had a lower frequency of laboratory test result abnormalities [35]. These data suggest that ESR may be related not only to the clinical activity of PMR but also to its severity. The need for corticosteroid therapy and the frequency of relapses were similar in patients with high and low ESRs [35]. Other studies have suggested that CRP levels are more sensitive than ESR levels in the assessment of disease activity in PMR [34].

Patients with temporal/giant cell arteritis almost always have elevated ESRs, with the mean ESR exceeding 90 mm/h [32]. Studies may have underestimated the rate of false-negative results [32]. This may occur because patients with a normal ESR are not likely to undergo temporal artery biopsy, which is the gold standard for establishing the diagnosis of temporal arteritis [32]. The false-positive rate of the ESR in patients who are suspected of having temporal arteritis is not known [32]. Therefore, the interpretation of an ESR depends on the clinician's estimate of the pretest probability for having temporal arteritis. When the clinical suspicion for temporal arteritis is low, a normal ESR reduces the probability of the disease to < 1% [32]. When clinical evidence supports the diagnosis of temporal arteritis, the disease may be present despite a normal ESR [32].

The American College of Rheumatology criteria for the classification of RA include an elevated ESR as one of 20 findings that may be present with the disease. An elevated ESR is not required for the diagnosis of RA. The ESR is a component of the remission criteria for RA and disease activity scores [36]. The role of ESR in distinguishing inflammatory articular disorders (eg, RA) from noninflammatory conditions (eg, osteo-arthritis) is questionable [4]. One study found that in patients with RA, only

50% had an ESR that exceeded 30 mm/h [4,32]. This rate was considerably higher than the rate in patients without RA with signs of osteoarthritis (14%). Therefore, an abnormal ESR may increase the probability of RA, but it is not diagnostic. Furthermore, a normal ESR provides little evidence for or against the diagnosis of RA. A careful history and physical examination is far more significant than an ESR in establishing the diagnosis.

The ESR can be helpful for measuring disease activity and response to treatment for some rheumatic diseases, including PMR, temporal arteritis, and RA, but the ESR level does not always reflect disease activity. Many patients started on corticosteroid therapy for polymyalgia rheumatic or temporal arteritis have an elevated ESR even when their clinical status has significantly improved [32]. Conversely, patients can have relapses of these conditions with a normal ESR level. Therefore, steroid therapy should not be based on the ESR level alone [32].

In RA, the ESR tends to reflect disease activity, but clinical symptoms and joint examination findings are considered more useful in assessing disease activity [32]. Although studies have correlated elevated ESRs with increased disease activity, evidence suggests that a significant proportion of patients in clinical remission may have an elevated ESR value and that a significant proportion of patients with a relapse may have an ESR <30 mm/h [32]. Therefore, although an increased ESR may be used as additional evidence of disease activity for RA, the ESR value alone should not be the reason for altering therapy [32].

The ESR is not helpful in following disease activity in SLE. The ESR often remains elevated even when the disease is controlled, usually due to a persistent polyclonal gammopathy [37].

C-Reactive Protein

Of the several acute-phase reactants, CRP is another commonly ordered test measuring systemic inflammation and is often compared with ESR. The CRP is named for its binding of the pneumococcal C-polysaccharide. The CRP is a rapid responder to inflammation and may be a better indicator of the acute-phase response during the first 24 hours in an inflammatory process than ESR [30]. CRP concentrations increase within 4 hours after an appropriate stimulus, peak within 24 to 72 hours, and may increase as much as 1000-fold [36]. They promptly return to normal when the underlying inflammation resolves. ESR levels rise over 24 to 48 hours and may not return to normal for weeks [38]. CRP levels can remain elevated in chronic inflammatory states, such as active RA. The CRP test is more expensive, less widely available, and more time-consuming to perform than the ESR. It usually needs to be sent to a well-equipped central laboratory, which may delay availability of results. CRP is directly measured and therefore is not affected by the variety of factors that influence ESR levels. CRP levels, as opposed to ESR levels, can be measured on stored or frozen sera. Many methods have been used to assay levels of CRP, and reporting units can vary. It is unclear whether these differences in laboratory techniques affect reported CRP levels.

Several conditions can cause elevated CRP levels. Examples of clinical conditions associated with CRP elevations in various degrees are shown in Table 6. CRP concentrations below 1 mg/dL but higher than seen in most normal subjects (0.2 mg/dL) have been found in patients with osteoarthritis. Such levels have been found to predict subsequent coronary events, indicating participation of inflammation in these disorders. Mild CRP elevations have been noted with increasing age [27].

Most rheumatic diseases, including RA, JCA, Reiter disease, ankylosing spondylitis, and psoriatic arthritis, are associated with high levels of CRP (1–10 mg/dL) when they are active [1]. However, studies have shown that CRP, unlike ESR, is usually not elevated in active SLE. Elevated CRP levels in patients with SLE are usually an indicator of infection rather than inflammation [1,27].

Whether CRP or ESR correlate better with disease activity in RA has been vigorously debated. The literature on the comparative value of the CRP and ESR tests is inconclusive, with studies suggesting that one or the other, or neither, is better [38,39]. CRP is used extensively in Europe, where it is believed to be the better test [38]. In the United States, 78% of rheumatologists use ESR to evaluate patients with RA, compared with 30% who use CRP [38]. CRP and ESR are often correlated, but in some situations CRP and ESR give different results. Although different studies suggest the superiority of one test over the other, the combined use of CRP and ESR most likely offers the most information [30].

TABLE 6.
Conditions Associated with Elevated C-Reactive Protein Levels

Normal or Insignificant Elevation (<1 mg/dL)	Moderate Elevation (1–10 mg/dL)	Marked Elevation (>10 mg/dL)
Vigorous exercise	Myocardial infarction	Acute bacterial infection (80% to 85%)
Common cold	Malignancies	Major trauma
Pregnancy	Pancreatitis	Systemic vasculitis
Gingivitis	Mucosal infection (bronchitis, cystitis)	
Cerebrovascular accident	Most rheumatic diseases	
Seizures		
Angina		

From Ballou S, Kushner I. Laboratory evaluation of inflammation. In: Ruddy S, Harris E, Sledge C, editors. Kelley's textbook of rheumatology. 6th edition. Philadelphia: WB Saunders; 2001; p. 698; with permission.

COMMONLY ASKED QUESTIONS REGARDING RHEUMATOLOGIC TESTING

When Is it Appropriate to Order an Antinuclear Antibody Test?

An ANA test is appropriate to order if the clinician has a reasonable clinical suspicion for SLE or another CTD based on the patient's history, physical findings, and results of other laboratory tests. Because of the large number of conditions associated with a positive ANA and the significant number of normal, healthy persons with a positive ANA, the ANA test should not be used for random screening for SLE or other CTDs. Ideally, clinicians use information collected from the history, physical examination, and previous laboratory work to estimate a pretest probability for disease. If patients have few signs or symptoms suggestive of disease, their pretest probability is low. A positive ANA in this case does little to increase the probability of disease and may lead to diagnostic confusion and unnecessary work-ups. On the other hand, if patients have signs and symptoms suggestive of disease, their pretest probability is higher. In this scenario, a positive ANA result can be helpful for supporting a diagnosis.

How Would You Evaluate an Unexplained Positive Antinuclear Antibody Test?

An ANA test should be used primarily as a confirmatory test when the physician strongly suspects SLE or another CTD. A positive ANA in isolation never makes a specific diagnosis. Many different rheumatologic conditions and nonrheumatologic conditions can cause a positive ANA, and a substantial number of normal individuals have a positive ANA test. Therefore, a positive ANA test alone does not necessitate further work-up unless the clinical context suggests the presence of SLE or another CTD. If the ANA titer is significantly elevated, it may be worthwhile to re-evaluate the titer in 6 to 12 months.

If an Antinuclear Antibody Test Result is Negative, Should the Test Be Repeated, or Should Other Tests Be Done?

Immediately repeating a negative ANA test is not necessary unless an error in testing is strongly suspected. Because systemic rheumatic diseases tend to evolve over time, if an ANA test is negative, it can be worthwhile to repeat the ANA test if the patient's clinical course develops new features consistent with a CTD.

Further antibody testing after a negative ANA test is generally not indicated. The use of HEp-2 cells as substrate has virtually eliminated false-negative ANA results. In rare instances where a CTD is strongly suspected, testing for specific autoantibodies (eg, anti-Ro, La, Jo-1, and phospholipids) and complement studies may be indicated (Box 3).

Box 3. Algorithm for the Use of ANA Testing

If clinician suspects SLE or other rheumatic disease: perform ANA test

ANA Negative
- No further autoantibody testing is indicated. Follow patient clinically and consider repeating testing if clinically indicated.
- If there is still high clinical suspicion for:
  SLE, consider anti-Ro/SS-A and anti-La/SS-B testing and complement studies
  Polymyositis/dermatomyositis, consider anti-Jo-1 testing
  Hypercoagulable state, consider antiphospholipid testing

ANA Positive
- If clinician suspects SLE but the diagnosis needs to be confirmed, consider testing for anti-dsDNA and anti-Sm.
- If SLE has been diagnosed and information is desired regarding prognosis or disease activity, consider testing for anti-dsDNA and anti-Ro/SS-A.
- If Sjögren's syndrome is suspected, consider testing for anti-Ro/SS-A and anti-La/SS-B.
- If polymyositis or dermatomyositis is suspected, consider testing for anti-Jo-1.
- If scleroderma is suspected, consider testing for anti-Scl-70 and anti-centromere.
- If drug-induced lupus is suspected, no further testing is indicated.
- If mixed connective tissue disease is suspected, consider testing for anti-U1 RNP.

Data from references 18–20.

Is It Helpful to Obtain Rheumatologic Tests to Rule Out Rheumatic Disease?

Although negative rheumatologic test results can be helpful and reassuring, the frequent occurrence of false-positive results renders these tests poor screening tools. The overuse and the nonselective ordering of rheumatologic tests have not only reduced the PPV of these tests but have led to unnecessary diagnoses, treatments, referrals, and work-ups. Thus, these tests should be ordered only to confirm a suspected diagnosis. Tests ordered in a setting of low pretest probability in an effort to rule out rheumatic disease will more likely add to diagnostic confusion rather than resolution. The American College of Rheumatology recommends ANA testing in patients who have unexplained signs or symptoms involving two or more organ systems [20]. Because of the high incidence of false-positive ANA titers, testing for ANA is not indicated in patients with isolated myalgias or arthralgias in the absence of other specific clinical and laboratory findings.

What Testing Should Be Ordered After a Positive Antinuclear Antibody Test Result?

Testing for specific autoantibodies after a positive ANA test result should be guided by the clinical circumstances and the suspicion of specific diseases (Box 3). The practice of "reflex" or "cascade" testing when an ANA test is positive, whereby large panels of tests are performed including various autoantibodies, is discouraged. This approach has little empirical evidence, can be costly, and can lead to erroneous diagnoses [10]. Guidelines from the College of American Pathologists suggest that for patients who meet the diagnostic criteria for SLE and have a positive ANA result, no further laboratory tests are necessary to make the diagnosis [10].

Which Is Better for Testing for Rheumatic Disease, C-Reactive Protein or Erythrocyte Sedimentation Rate? When Should Either One Be Ordered?

Both tests measure components of the acute phase response and are useful for measuring generalized inflammation. The ESR is measured indirectly and is affected by multiple variables (Table 5). It is therefore less precise. However, it is inexpensive and easy to perform. The CRP is directly measured and is unaffected by the factors influencing the ESR. It rises more quickly and falls more rapidly than the ESR. The CRP is more costly, difficult to perform, and less available. Although both tests can be helpful for assessing the degree of inflammation and disease activity in rheumatic conditions, their results do not always agree. This discordance can be attributed to the variables affecting ESR levels and the different sensitivities of each test to various conditions. Many authors seem to agree that information gathered from both tests may be more helpful than either alone. The literature expresses significant contention regarding which is the better test for different rheumatic conditions.

What Do You Do when a Patient Has an Elevated Erythrocyte Sedimentation Rate?

A clinician can perform a history, physical examination, and routine screening laboratory tests (complete blood count, chemistries, liver enzymes, and urinalysis) to explain an elevated ESR. Although many clinicians find an unexplained elevated ESR difficult to ignore, most of these patients do not have serious disease [32]. Most unexplained increases in ESR are transitory. If there is no obvious cause for the elevated ESR, recheck it in 1 to 3 months. The ESR level in up to 80% of patients normalizes with that time [26,32]. Follow patients for development of other signs or symptoms of disease if ESR remains elevated [26]. Consider checking a serum protein electrophoresis to rule out myeloma or polyclonal gammopathy and checking a CRP for additional evidence of an activated acute phase response [26].

Key Points

- The results of common rheumatologic laboratory tests play an important part in the diagnosis and management of rheumatic diseases.
- Rheumatologic test results can often be ambiguous and can sometimes be misleading, particularly in primary care settings.
- Test results should be interpretted in a clinical context, which includes information derived from the history, physical examination, basic laboratory tests, radiographic and other imaging studies, and synovial fluid analysis.
- Serum rheumatologic tests are most useful for confirming a clinically suspected diagnosis.
- Because there is a high incidence of false-positive results in the general population, these tests have limited clinical utility when there is a low pretest probability.
- Recognizing the limitations of rheumatologic test may improve their utility by encouraging more selective testing and more cautious interpretation of test results.

References

[1] Pincus T. Laboratory tests in rheumatic disorders. In: Klippel J, Dieppe P, editors. Rheumatology. 2nd edition. Philadelphia: Mosby; 1998.
[2] Kavanaugh A, Tomar R, Reveille J, et al. Guidelines for clinical use of the antinuclear antibody test and tests for specific autoantibodies to nuclear antigens. Arch Pathol Lab Med 2000;124:71–81.
[3] Suarez-Almazor M, Gonzalez-Lopez L, Gamez-Nava I, et al. Utilization and predictive value of laboratory tests in patients referred to rheumatologists by primary care physicians. J Rheumatol 1998;25:1980–5.
[4] Snow C. Laboratory testing for musculoskeletal diseases. In: Harris E, Genovese M, editors. Primary care rheumatology. Philadelphia: W.B. Saunders Company; 2000.
[5] Shmerling R, Delbanco T. The rheumatoid factor: an analysis of clinical utility. Am J Med 1991;91:528–34.
[6] Lane S. Clinical utility of common serum rheumatologic tests. Am Fam Physician 2002;65:1073–80.
[7] Egner W. The use of laboratory tests in the diagnosis of SLE. J Clin Pathol 2000;53: 424–32.
[8] Solomon D, Kavanaugh A, Schur P, the American College of Rheumatology Ad Hoc Committee on Immunologic Testing Guidelines. Evidence-Based guidelines for the use of immunologic tests: anti nuclear antibody testing. Arthritis Rheum 2002;47:434–44.
[9] Feigenbaum P, Medsger T, Kraines R, et al. The variability of immunologic laboratory tests. J Rheumatol 1982;9:408–14.
[10] Kavanaugh A, Solomon D, Schur P, et al. Guidelines for immunologic laboratory testing in the rheumatic diseases: an introduction. Arthritis Rheum 2002;47:429–33.
[11] Arnett F, Edworthy S, Bloch D, et al. The American Rheumatism Association 1987 revised criteria for the classification of rheumatoid arthritis. Arthritis Rheum 1988;31: 315–24.
[12] Wolfe F, Cathey M, Roberts F. The latex test revisited: rheumatoid factor testing in 8,287 rheumatic disease patients. Arthritis Rheum 1991;34:951–60.
[13] Shmerling R, Delbanco T. How useful is the rheumatoid factor? An analysis of sensitivity, specificity, and predictive value. Arch Intern Med 1992;152:2417–20.

[14] Carson D. Rheumatoid factor. In: Kelley W, Harris E, Ruddy S, Sledge C, editors. Sledge Kelley's textbook of rheumatology. 4th edition. Philadelphia: WB Saunders; 1993. p. 155–63.

[15] Tighe H, Carson D. Rheumatoid factor. In: Ruddy S, Harris E, Sledge C, editors. Kelley's textbook of rheumatology. 6th edition. Philadelphia: WB Saunders; 2001. p. 151–60.

[16] Keren D. Antinuclear antibody testing. Clin Lab Med 2002;22:447–74.

[17] Moder K. Use and interpretation of rheumatologic tests: a guide for clinicians. Mayo Clin Proc 1996;71:391–6.

[18] Peng S, Craft J. Antinuclear antibodies. In: Ruddy S, Harris E, Sledge C, editors. Kelley's textbook of rheumatology. 6th edition. Philadelphia: WB Saunders; 2001. p. 161–74.

[19] Craft J, Hardin J. Antinuclear antibodies. In: Kelley W, Harris E, Ruddy S, Sledge C, editors. Kelley's textbook of rheumatology. 4th edition. Philadelphia: WB Saunders; 1993. p. 164–87.

[20] Gladman D, Urowitz M, Esdaile J, et al. American College of Rheumatology Ad Hoc Committee on Systemic Lupus Erythematosus Guidelines. Guidelines for referral and management of systemic lupus erythematosus in adults. Arthitis Rheum 1999;42: 1785–96.

[21] Tan E, Cohen A, Fries J, et al. The 1982 revised criteria for the classification of systemic lupus erythematosus. Arthritis Rheum 1982;25:1271–7.

[22] Hochberg M. Updating the American College of Rheumatology revised criteria for the classification of systemic lupus erythematosus [letter] Arthritis Rheum 1997;40: 1725.

[23] Tan E, Feltkamp W, Smolen J, et al. Range of antinuclear antibodies in "healthy" individuals. Arthritis Rheum 1997;40:1601–11.

[24] Tozzoli R, Bizzaro N, Tonutti E, et al. Guidelines for the laboratory use of autoantibody tests in the diagnosis and monitoring of autoimmune rheumatic diseases. Am J Clin Pathol 2002;117:316–24.

[25] Homburger H. Laboratory medicine and pathology: cascade testing for autoantibodies in connective tissue diseases. Mayo Clin Proc 1995;70:183–4.

[26] Hobbs K. Laboratory evaluation. In: West S, editor. Rheumatology secrets. 2nd edition. Philadelphia: Hanley & Belfus; 2002. p. 52–63.

[27] Ballou S, Kushner I. Laboratory evaluation of inflammation. In: Ruddy S, Harris E, Sledge C, editors. Kelley's textbook of rheumatology. 6th edition. Philadelphia: WB Saunders; 2001. p. 697–703.

[28] Ward M. Laboratory testing for systemic rheumatic diseases. Postgrad Med 1998;103: 93–100.

[29] Wolfe F, Hawley D. The longterm outcomes of rheumatoid arthritis: work disability: a prospective 18 year study of 823 patients. J Rheumatol 1998;25:2108–17.

[30] Otterness I. The value of C-reactive protein measurement in rheumatoid arthritis. Semin Arthritis Rheum 1994;24:91–104.

[31] Dawes P, Fowler S, Fisher C, et al. Rheumatoid arthritis: treatment which controls the C-reactive protein and erythrocyte sedimentation rate reduces radiological progression. Br J Rheumatol 1986;25:44–9.

[32] Sox H, Liang M. The erythrocyte sedimentation rate: guidelines for rational use. Ann Intern Med 1986;104:515–23.

[33] Brigden M. Clinical utility of the erythrocyte sedimentation rate. Am Fam Physician 1999;60:1443–50.

[34] Cantini F, Salvarani C, Olivieri I. Erythrocyte sedimentation rate and C-reactive protein in the diagnosis of polymyalgia rheumatica. Ann Intern Med 1998;128:873–4.

[35] Gonzalez-Gay M, Rodriguez-Valverde V, Blanco R, et al. Polymyalgia rheumatica without significantly increased erythrocyte sedimentation rate. Arch Intern Med 1997;157: 317–20.

[36] Paulus H, Brahn E. Is erythrocyte sedimentation rate the preferable measure of the acutephase response in rheumatoid arthritis? J Rheumatol 2004;31:838–40.

[37] Kotzin B. Systemic lupus erythematosus. In: West S, editor. Rheumatology secrets. 2nd edition. Philadelphia: Hanley & Belfus; 2002. p. 128–47.

[38] Wolfe F. Comparative usefullness of C-reactive protein and erythrocyte sedimentation rate in patients with rheumatoid arthritis. J Rheumatol 1997;24:1477–85.

[39] Ward M. Relative sensitivity to change of the erythrocyte sedimentation rate and serum C-reactive protein concentration in rheumatoid arthritis. J Rheumatol 2004;31:884–93.
[40] Hanly J. Antiphospholipid syndrome: an overview. CMAJ 2003;168:1675–82.
[41] Bottiger L, Svedberg C. Normal erythrocyte sedimentation rate and age. BMJ 1967;2: 85–7.

Address reprint requests to

Brooke Salzman, MD
Department of Family Medicine
Thomas Jefferson University
1015 Walnut Street, Suite 401
Philadelphia, PA 19107

e-mail: brookesalzman@comcast.net

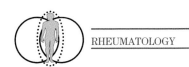
RHEUMATOLOGY   1522–5720/05 $15.00 + .00

JOINT AND SOFT TISSUE INJECTIONS IN PRIMARY CARE

Peter J. Carek, MD, MS, and Melissa H. Hunter, MD

In 1951, Hollander introduced local corticosteroid injection therapy for the treatment of inflammatory arthritis [1]. Since that time, aspiration of synovial fluid and injection of joints, bursae, tendon sheaths, and soft tissues are frequently used diagnostic and therapeutic skills for many physicians practicing in the outpatient setting. In one study, nearly 90% of family physicians reported performing joint aspiration and injection at least once per month [2].

Despite the common use of this procedure, the reported medical benefits of intra-articular injection are inconsistent and seem to be affected by numerous variables, including diagnosis, site of injection, medications used, and additional incorporated therapies. For instance, intra-articular steroid injections have produced clinically and statistically significant reduction in osteoarthritic knee pain 1 week after injection [3]. In a meta-analysis, Arroll [4] determined that evidence supports short-term (up to 2 weeks) improvement in symptoms of osteoarthritis of the knee after intra-articular corticosteroid injection. The beneficial effect has been found to last for 3 to 4 weeks. Local corticosteroid injection as treatment for flexor tenosynovitis was found to be 90% effective in relieving symptoms, and serious adverse effects were avoided if guidelines were followed [5].

Corticosteroid injections have not been shown to provide clear benefit for shoulder pain [6]. The benefits of treating other common conditions with intra-articular or soft tissue injection require additional study. Other issues that remain to be clarified include whether accuracy of needle placement, anatomic site, frequency, dose, and type of corticosteroid influences efficacy. The efficacy of other conditions commonly treated with corticosteroid injection (eg, lateral epicondylitis, plantar fascitis, etc.) is not well known.

From the Department of Family Medicine, Medical University of South Carolina, Charleston, South Carolina

INDICATIONS

Aspiration of synovial fluid is indicated to further evaluate a spontaneous, unexplained joint effusion with or without associated trauma if the diagnosis is uncertain. Analysis of the synovial fluid is required if septic arthritis is suspected. Joint aspiration can limit joint damage from an infectious process and can provide relief from a large effusion. Depending on the joint, aspiration of large amounts of synovial fluid may occur. The amount of synovial fluid aspirated from a knee may range from 50 to 100 mL.

Physical characteristics (eg, color, clarity, and viscosity), white blood cell (WBC) count and differential, presence of crystals (polarized light), and microbiology (Gram stain, bacterial culture) are the most useful studies in analyzing synovial fluid [7]. Data support the performance of synovial fluid WBC count with differential, Gram stain and culture, and examination of crystals by polarizing microscopy [8]. Additional studies are usually not warranted and are rarely beneficial.

Based upon the findings of the laboratory studies, the synovial fluid can be classified (eg, as noninflammatory, inflammatory, septic, or hemorrhagic), and a differential diagnosis can be delineated (Tables 1 and 2) [9]. The presumptive diagnosis of a septic arthritis and a differentiation between a noninflammatory and an inflammatory condition can be established.

Injection of joints and soft tissues is used for the diagnosis and treatment of numerous musculoskeletal diagnoses (Box 1) [10,11]. The injection of a local anesthetic may assist in the confirmation of a diagnosis if symptom relief occurs. For example, shoulder impingement syndrome is frequently evaluated by injecting short-acting anesthetic into the subacromial space and monitoring for improvement or resolution of symptoms.

CONTRAINDICATIONS

Several absolute and relative contraindications for joint and soft tissue injections exist (Box 2) [11–13]. In general, these contraindications are recommendations and should be used on an individual basis in determining an effective yet safe treatment plan for each patient. For instance, although suspected septic arthritis is an absolute contraindication for joint injection, a suspected septic arthritis is an indication for joint aspiration.

Additional precautions should be considered. If an underlying fracture is possible, plain radiographs should be considered before aspiration and injection of a joint. In the primary care setting, injection of musculotendinous sites at high risk for rupture (eg, Achilles tendon, patella tendon) is usually not indicated.

GENERAL TECHNIQUE

For joint and soft tissue injections, the materials, equipment, and pharmacologic agents need to be selected. In addition, informed consent

TABLE 1.
Classes of Synovial Fluid Based upon Laboratory Studies

	Class I (noninflammatory)	Class II (inflammatory)	Class III (septic)	Class IV (hemorrhagic)
Color	Clear/yellow	Yellow/white	Yellow/white	Red
Clarity	Transparent	Translucent/opaque	Opaque	Opaque
Viscosity	High	Variable	Low	Not applicable
Mucin clot	Firm	Variable	Friable	Not applicable
WBC count	<2000	2000–100,000	>100,000	Not applicable
Differential	<25% PMNs	>50% PMNs	>95% PMNs	Not applicable
Culture	Negative	Negative	Positive	Variable

Abbreviation: PMN, polymorphonuclear leukocyte.

Data from Klippel JH, Weyand CM, Crofford LH, et al, editors. Primer on the rheumatic diseases. 12th edition. Atlanta (GA): Arthritis Foundation; 2001. p. 140–3.

TABLE 2.
Differential Diagnosis Based upon Synovial Class

Class I	Class II	Class III	Class IV
Osteoarthritis	Rheumatoid arthritis	Bacterial	Trauma
Traumatic	SLE	arthritis	Pigmented
arthritis	Scleroderma		villonodular
Osteonecrosis	Systemic necrotizing		synovitis
Charcot's	vasculitides		Tuberculosis
arthropathy	Polychondritis		Tumor
	Gout		Coagulopathy
	CPPD deposition disease		Charcot
	Hydroxyapatite deposition		arthropathy
	Juvenile rheumatoid arthritis		
	Seronegative		
	spondyloarthopathies		
	Psoriatic arthritis		
	Reactive arthritis		
	CIBD		
	Hypogammaglobulinemia		
	Sarcoidosis		
	Rheumatic fever		
	Indolent/low virulence infections		
	(viral, mycobacterial, fungal,		
	Whipple disease, Lyme		
	arthritis)		

Abbreviations: CIBD, chronic inflammatory bowel disease; SLE, systemic lupus erythematosus.

Data from Klippel JH, Weyand CM, Crofford LH, et al, editors. Primer on the rheumatic diseases. 12th edition. Atlanta (GA): Arthritis Foundation; 2001. p. 140–3.

explaining the procedure, potential risks, and complications and side effects should be obtained from the patient before the injection. Information about medication allergies or adverse reaction to previous injection should be elicited.

Materials and Equipment

All joint and soft tissue injections should be performed using gloves. Typically, nonsterile gloves are appropriate for joint or soft tissue injections as long as the site is not handled after aseptic preparation and before the completion of the procedure. If the site is to be handled, then sterile gloves are required. Other equipment necessary for joint and soft tissue injection should be made readily available before the procedure (Box 3).

**Box 1. Conditions Often Treated with Local
Injection Therapy [10,11]**

Articular conditions
- Rheumatoid arthritis
- Seronegative spondyloarthropathies
- Ankylosing spondylitis
- Arthritis associated with inflammatory bowel disease
- Psoriasis
- Reiter syndrome
- Crystal-induced arthritis
- Gout
- Pseudogout
- Osteoarthritis (acute exacerbation)

Nonarticular disorders
- Fibrositis
- Bursitis
  Subacromial
  Trochanteric
  Anserine
  Prepatellar
- Tenosynovitis/tendonitis
  De Quervain disease
  Stenosing tenosynovitis (trigger finger)
  Bicipital
  Lateral epicondylitis (tennis elbow)
  Medial epicondylitis (golfer's elbow)
  Plantar fasciitis
- Neuritis
  Carpal tunnel syndrome
  Tarsal tunnel syndrome

Pharmacologic Agents

Corticosteroids

Corticosteroids are believed to modify the local inflammatory response through stabilization of lysosomal membranes, inhibition of cellular metabolism (eg, neutrophil chemotaxis and function), inhibition of polymorphonuclear leukocyte membrane microtubular function, and establishment of decreased local synovial permeability. These corticosteroids are felt to increase the viscosity of synovial fluid, alter production of hyaluronic acid synthesis, and change synovial fluid leukocyte activity [14]. Because intra-articular steroid administration can maximize local benefits and minimize systemic adverse effects, patients can often obtain significant relief from acute exacerbations of osteoarthritis.

Although many preparations are available for joint and soft tissue injections, corticosteroids differ with respect to potency, solubility, and

---

Box 2. Contraindications to Joint Injections [11–13]

- Overlying cellulitis*
- Severe coagulopathy
- Anticoagulant therapy
- Septic effusion
- More than three injections per year in a weight-bearing joint
- Lack of response after two to four injections
- Bacteremia*
- Unstable joints
- Inaccessible joints (eg, facet joints of spine)
- Joint prosthesis*
- Evidence of surrounding osteoporosis
- Recent intra-articular joint osteoporosis
- History of allergy or anaphylaxis to injectable pharmaceuticals

　*Absolute contraindications.

---

relative duration of action. Potency of individual agents is generally measured against hydrocortisone and ranges from low-potency, short-acting agents (eg, cortisone) to high-potency, longer-acting agents (eg, betamethasone) (Table 3).

Few studies have investigated the duration of action of corticosteroid agents in joints or soft tissues. In general, the duration of effect is inversely related to the solubility of the therapeutic agent (ie, less soluble agents remain in the joint or area longer and provide a more prolonged effect). For instance, suspensions are considered to be longer acting, whereas solutions are shorter acting, less irritating to the joint space, and less likely to produce a postinjection flare.

Box 3. Equipment Commonly Used for Joint or Soft Tissue Injections

- Alcohol wipes
- Povidone-iodine wipes
- Sterile and nonsterile gloves
- Sterile drapes
- 25- to 30-gauge, 0.5- to 1.0-inch needle (local skin anesthesia)
- 22- to 25-gauge, 1.0- to 1.5-inch needle (intra-articular injections)
- 1 mL to 10 mL syringe. A larger syringe may be required for aspiration of a large joint (eg, the knee).
- Local anesthetic
- Corticosteroid preparation
- Adhesive bandage dressing

TABLE 3.
Relative Potency of Corticosteroid Preparations

Corticosteroid	Relative Anti-inflammatory Potency	Approximate Equivalent Dose (mg)
Short-acting preparations		
Cortisone	0.8	25
Hydrocortisone	1.0	20
Intermediate-acting preparations		
Prednisone	4	5
Methylprednisolone acetate (Depo-Medrol)	5	4
Long-acting preparations		
Dexamethasone sodium phosphate (Decadron)	25	0.6
Betamethasone (Celestone Soluspan)	25	0.6

Data from Cardone DA, Tallia AF. Joint and soft tissue injection. Am Fam Physician 2002; 66:283–8.

Agents with low solubility should be used primarily for intra-articular therapy and should be avoided in soft tissues due to the increased risk of soft tissue atrophy from prolonged local corticosteroid action. Methylprednisolone is often the agent of choice for soft tissue injections.

The dosage of each individual corticosteroid is site-dependent, with larger joints requiring higher doses. General dosing guidelines for soft tissue and relative joint sizes are provided in Table 4.

TABLE 4.
Dosages of Corticosteroid Preparations

Corticosteroid	Preparation Strength (mg/mL)	Common dosage for site (mg)		
		Tendon Sheaths and Bursae	Small Joints	Large Joints
Hydrocortisone	25,50	8–40	10–25	50–125
Methylprednisolone (Depo-Medrol)	20,40,80	4–10	2–5	10–25
Betamethasone (Celestone Soluspan)	6	1.5–3.0	0.8–1.0	2–4

Data from Refs. [10,11,13].

Hyaluronic Acid

Intra-articular injection of hyaluronic acid is used to treat the pain associated with osteoarthritis of the knee. The rationale for the use of hyalurons therapeutically is based on observations that hyaluronic acid is an important component of the synovial fluid that acts as a cushion and lubricant for the joint and serves as a major component of the extracellular matrix of the cartilage, helping to enhance the ability of cartilage to resist shear and maintain a resiliency to compression [15]. Intra-articular injection of hyaluronic acid for the treatment of osteoarthritis of the knee has been found to be safe and effective (grade of recommendation: A) [16,17]. No differences were detected between patients treated for osteoarthritis of the knee with intra-articular injections of hyaluronic acid and patients treated with corticosteroid with respect to pain relief or function at 6 months of follow-up [18].

Intra-articular injection of hyaluronic acid is indicated for the treatment of pain in osteoarthritis of the knee in patients who have failed to respond adequately to conservative, nonpharmacologic therapy and simple analgesics. Three to five injections are given in weekly intervals. Injection site pain and local purities are the most common adverse effects.

Anesthetics

For intra-articular or soft tissue injections, an anesthetic is mixed with the corticosteroid. This procedure facilitates the injection process, often providing temporary analgesia, confirming delivery of the medication to the appropriate site, and diluting the crystalline suspension, thus providing better diffusion of medication throughout the injected region. When mixing anesthetics and corticosteroids, the presence of preservatives such as phenols and parabens should raise some concern regarding possible precipitation of the corticosteroid preparation. If possible, preservative-free anesthetic solutions should be used.

Lidocaine. With respect to the use of anesthetic agents, a preparation of 1% lidocaine is frequently used due to its rapid onset of activity in the injected region. Because of its short half-life, lidocaine's duration of effect is short (ie, 1–2 hours) [19].

Bupivacaine. When longer local analgesia is desired, the use of an agent such as bupivacaine is preferable. Bupivacaine has a longer onset of than lidocaine (ie, 2–10 minutes) and a longer duration of effect (3–6 hours). Bupivacaine is available in solution strengths ranging from 0.25% to 0.75%. If precipitation of corticosteroid is a concern, preservative-free solutions of bupivacaine are available.

Site Preparation

The use of aseptic technique minimizes the risk of infection into a joint or soft tissue. The injection site can be clearly identified by an imprint using the blunt end of a pen or by a deeply embedded fingernail. Provadine iodine is applied to the area and allowed to dry for greatest aseptic effect. The immediate injection site can then be cleaned with a sterile alcohol swab. The use of local anesthetic in the skin and subcutaneous tissues overlying the injection site is optional. Spraying sterile ethyl chloride onto the skin, applying ice to the area for 5 to 10 minutes, or firmly pinching the skin for several seconds are alternatives to reduce the discomfort associated with injection.

For soft tissue injections, placement of the corticosteroid into the skin or subcutaneous tissue should be avoided to minimize the risk of localized skin atrophy. The corticosteroid should not be injected directly into a tendon or ligament to avoid possible rupture of these structures. The needle should be repositioned if resistance is encountered during steroid injection. Finally, aspiration should be attempted before the infiltration of a structure to avoid intravascular deposition of medication.

Postinjection Care

After injection, passive and active range of motion of the joint may assist in promoting corticosteroid distribution throughout the joint space. Pain relief after joint or soft tissue injection with a local anesthetic may indicate that the appropriate structure was infiltrated.

Although use of corticosteroid injections for soft tissue and joints may provide short-term pain relief for many patients, some caveats should be observed with respect to reinjection of the same anatomic area. A patient's response to previous injections is important when making a decision to proceed with reinjection of the same area. For patients who have received no symptom relief or functional improvement after two injections, the likelihood for pain relief with subsequent injections is low [20].

If a therapeutic effect from injections is achieved, caution should be undertaken to avoid a polyinjection syndrome (ie, no more than three to four injections per year is recommended in large weight-bearing joints). This precaution helps to avoid joint instability from osteonecrosis of juxta-articular bone and weakening of capsular ligaments [20,21]. Repeat injections of the same area should occur no more than 6 to 12 weeks apart. Injecting several large joints simultaneously (or no more than three in a month) should be avoided due to the increased risk of hypothalamic-pituitary-adrenal suppression and other adverse effects [22]. Therapeutic injection of large or weight-bearing joint should not be performed more than three times per year, and individual injections should be separated by 6 weeks or more.

COMPLICATIONS

Intra- and periarticular steroid injections have been found to be safe and to have low complication rates if performed while taking adequate precautions (Table 5) [22,23]. Postinjection infection rates of 1:16,000 to

TABLE 5.
Adverse Effects of Local Corticosteroid Therapy

Complications	Estimated Prevalence
Postinjection flare	2–5%
Steroid arthropathy	0.8%
Tendon rupture	<1%
Facial flushing	<1%
Skin atrophy, depigmentation	<1%
Iatrogenic infectious arthritis	<0.001% to 0.072%
Transient paresis of injected extremity	Rare
Hypersensitivity reaction	Rare
Asymptomatic pericapsular calcification	43%
Acceleration of cartilage attrition	Unknown

Adapted from Gray RG, Gottlieb NL. Intra-articular corticosteroids: an updated assessment. Clin Orthop 1983;177:235–63.

1–2:150,000 have been cited [20,24]. In a study of the use of aseptic technique without sterile gloves or drapes, only 18 of 250,000 (0.072%) injections were complicated by infection [10]. When the injection site was prepared with an alcohol solution and disposable needles and syringes were used, the infection rate was found to be 0.0001% [25]. Pal [26] estimated the risk of bacterial arthritis after intra-articular corticosteroid injection to be low (4.6:100,000 injections). In a survey of orthopedic surgeons, rheumatologists, and general practitioners, Charalambous [27] found that septic arthritis after an intra-articular steroid injection of the knee is probably rare. In this study, 57.6% of the respondents used alcohol swabs to clean the skin, and the remaining 42.4% used chlorhexidine and Betadine.

Trauma to surrounding anatomic structures or tissue such as ligaments, tendons, neurovascular bundles, or articular cartilage may occur, although the incidence has not been frequently reported. Injury to these structures can be avoided with the use of proper injection technique. Achilles tendon rupture has been reported after local corticosteroid administration.

Complications or adverse reactions to the medications are possible. Allergic reactions to the anesthetic or preservatives in the injected solution may occur. A crystal-induced synovitis or postinjection steroid flare has been reported and usually occurs within 1 to 2 days after the injection. This condition is usually self-limiting and responds to ice.

The corticosteroid may produce untoward effects, such as the exacerbation of a chronic condition or an alteration in the structure of localized tissue. Although rarely reported and the specific incidence unknown, episodes of elevated plasma glucose levels have been reported in individuals with diabetes mellitus who have received local corticosteroid injections [28]. Subcutaneous atrophy of tissue can occur when the corticosteroid is injected less than 5 mm beneath the skin surface. Boston [29] reported significant atrophy in 13% of knees injected locally at the tibial tubercle with a corticosteroid. If the corticosteroid is injected into an early septic joint, acceleration of the infection may occur. Weakening of a large tendon (eg, Achilles and patella) can cause damage to cartilage, and the development of localized osteoporosis may be a concern.

SPECIFIC INJECTIONS BY SITE

The medical benefits of intra-articular and soft tissue injection are inconsistent and seem to be affected by numerous variables, including diagnosis, site of injection, medications used, and additional incorporated therapies. As such, an overall recommendation for their use cannot be provided based upon current literature. Therefore, an evidence-based recommendation (Table 6) and injection technique for individual sites are provided.

Shoulder

Corticosteroid injection of the shoulder may be used for treatment of such conditions as subacromial bursitis, rotator cuff tendonitis, adhesive capsulitis, and biceps tendonitis (grade of recommendation: D). The evidence in favor of the efficacy of steroid injections for shoulder disorders is scarce [30]. As noted by Buchbinder [6], the overall evidence to guide the use of corticosteroid injections for shoulder pain is inconsistent. The number, site, and dosage of injections varied widely between the studies reviewed. Subacromial corticosteroid injection for rotator cuff disease

TABLE 6.
Grades of Recommendations for Selected Injections

Injection Site/Diagnosis	Grade of Recommendation
Shoulder (subacromial bursitis, rotator cuff tendonitis, adhesive capsulitis, and biceps tendonitis)	D
Lateral epicondylitis	A
Medial epicondylitis	D
Trigger finger	C
DeQuervain tenosynovitis	C
Carpal tunnel	A
Trochanteric bursitis	C
Knee (osteoarthritis, bursitis)	A
Plantar fasciitis	D

may be beneficial, although the effect may be small and not well maintained.

Subacromial Bursa

The subacromial bursa can be entered by a lateral or posterior approach (Fig. 1). To maximize the potential space under the acromion process, the patient should sit with his shoulder in neutral position and his

FIGURE 1.
(A–C) The lateral and posterior location and approach to the subacromial injection.

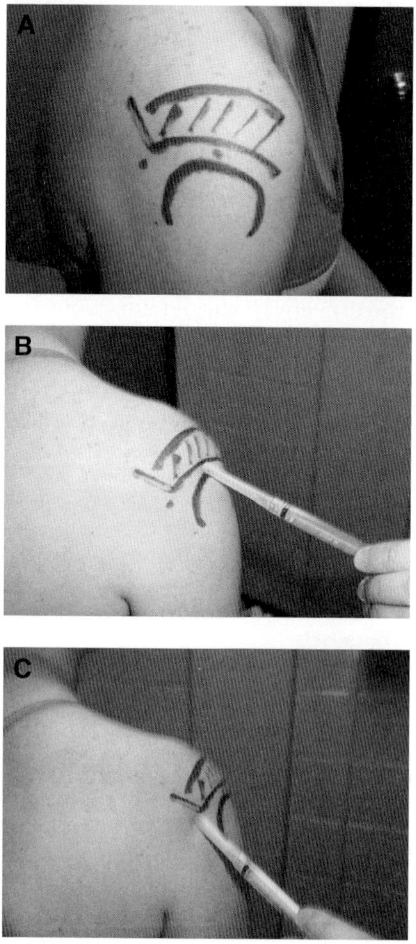

hands on his lap. Mild inferior traction of the humerus can be applied. With the lateral approach, the needle is inserted 1 to 2 cm below the lower edge of the acromion through the deltoid with a slightly superior approach. For the posterior approach, the needle is inserted below the inferior edge of the acromion as it intersects with the scapular spine.

Glenohumeral Joint

The needle is inserted anteriorly at a point 1 cm inferior and 1 to 2 cm lateral to the coracoid process. The needle is direct posteriorly.

Biceps Tendon

The tendon sheath is injected by inserting the needle parallel to the tendon near the bicipital groove, usually at the point of most tenderness.

Elbow

Corticosteroid injection of the elbow is indicated in the management of lateral epicondylitis (grade of recommendation: A) and medial epicondylitis (grade of recommendation: D). In a systematic review of randomized clinical trials, corticosteroid injections for lateral epicondylitis seem to be relatively safe and seem to be effective in short-term treatment (2–6 weeks) [31]. Corticosteroid injections were significantly better than all other therapy options for all outcome measures at 6 weeks, whereas physiotherapy provided the best results for these same measures at 52 weeks [32]. The recurrence rate in the injection group was high.

The response to corticosteroid injection may provide prognostic information. Patients who achieved pain control after a single cortisone injection successfully avoided surgery 88% of the time, whereas those requiring multiple injections avoided surgery only 44% of the time [33]. Based upon these findings, a single corticosteroid injection for lateral epicondylitis could be attempted as part of the initial treatment plan.

Lateral Epicondyle

The area of greatest discomfort is determined (Fig. 2). The origin of the extensor carpi radialis brevis is identified by having the patient extend the middle finger against resistance as the epicondylar area is palpated. The needle is inserted into the site of greatest discomfort.

Medial Epicondyle

The needle is inserted into the area of greatest discomfort on the medical epicondyle. During this injection, the ulnar nerve located on the poster aspect of the medical epicondyle needs to be avoided.

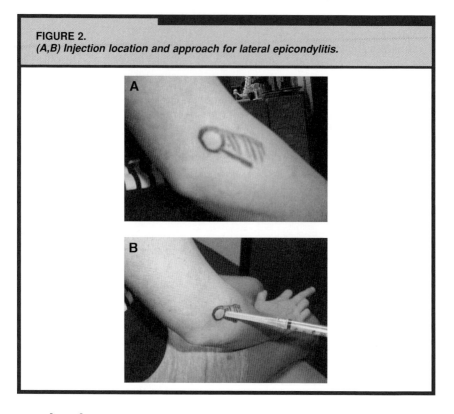

FIGURE 2.
(A,B) Injection location and approach for lateral epicondylitis.

Hand and Wrist

Trigger Finger

Corticosteroid injection seems to be an effective treatment option for trigger finger (grade of recommendation: C). Up to 75% of triggering fingers and thumbs demonstrated improvement or resolution with corticosteroid injections [34]. In another study, a single injection cured 64% of patients with primary trigger finger [35].

At the level of the stenosis (usually just proximal to the proximal crease of the affected digit), the needle is directed proximally toward the center of the palm at a 30° to 45° angle (Fig. 3). If active flexion of the tendon by the patient causes movement of the needle and syringe, the needle should be repositioned to avoid injecting the tendons.

De Quervain Tenosynovitis

De Quervain tenosynovitis can be effectively treated with corticosteroid injections (grade of recommendation: C). In a group of patients with moderate or severe symptoms, 76% were completely relieved, and 7% were improved after treatment with local corticosteroid injection [36].

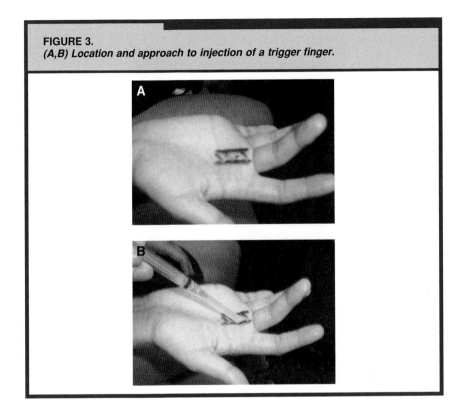

FIGURE 3.
(A,B) Location and approach to injection of a trigger finger.

The area of greatest discomfort in the area of the extensor pollicis brevis and abductor pollicis longus tendons is determined. The affected tendon sheaths are entered and injected. As with trigger finger injection, the tendon can be avoided by having the patient abduct and extend the thumb and determine any movement of the needle. If it moves, the needle needs to be repositioned.

Carpal Tunnel

For carpal tunnel syndrome, corticosteroid injection provides temporary, short-term improvement (grade of recommendation: A). As noted by Marshall [37] in a review of randomized trials, local corticosteroid injection for carpal tunnel syndrome provided greater clinical improvement in symptoms 1 month after injection compared with placebo. Local corticosteroid injection did not provide improved clinical outcome compared with anti-inflammatory treatment or splinting after 8 weeks.

For local carpal tunnel injection, the needle is inserted just ulnar to the palmaris longus tendon (or flexor carpi radialis if the palmaris longus is absent) at the level of the distal wrist crease and directed 45° distally. This approach allows for entry into the carpal tunnel space through the overlying retinaculum.

Hip

Trochanteric Bursa

Corticosteroid injection is an effective option for the treatment of trochanteric bursitis (grade of recommendation: C). In a series of 36 cases of simple trochanteric bursitis, Ege [38] reported that one or two local corticosteroid injections gave excellent response in two thirds and improvement in the remaining cases. One fourth of the cases relapsed within 2 years.

The needle is introduced over the site of greatest discomfort over the greater trochanter. The needle is inserted to the level of the periosteum and is withdrawn slightly. In a large or obese individual, a 3-cm spinal needle may be required to reach the periosteum and the bursa.

Knee

Injections of the knee are recommended for the treatment of such conditions as osteoarthritis and bursitis (grade of recommendation: A). Intra-articular steroid injection produces a clinically and statistically significant reduction in osteoarthritic knee pain 1 week after injection [3]. In a meta-analysis, Arroll [4] determined that evidence from randomized controlled trials supports short-term (up to 2 weeks) improvement in symptoms of osteoarthritis of the knee after intra-articular corticosteroid injection. No differences were detected between patients treated for osteoarthritis of the knee with intra-articular injections of hyaluronic acid and those treated with corticosteroid with respect to pain relief or function at 6 months of follow-up [18]. No deleterious effects of the long-term administration of intra-articular steroids on the anatomic structure of the knee have been noted [39].

Intra-articular Space

Two techniques may be used to reach the intra-articular space of the knee. With the patient in a supine position, a medial or lateral approach may used. For the lateral approach, the insertion point is located just lateral to the superolateral portion of the patella (1 cm above and 1 cm lateral to the superior lateral aspect of the patella) with the needle directed 45° distally and posteriorly to pass underneath the patella. With the patient sitting with the knee flexed 90°, the intra-articular space may be reached by inserting the needle immediately medial or lateral to the patella tendon just superior to the tibial plateau and directing it toward the middle of the knee (Fig. 4).

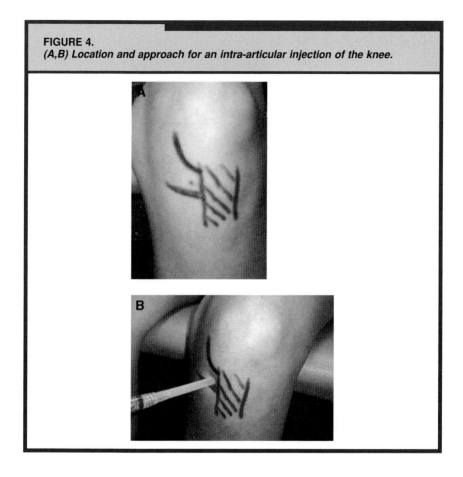

FIGURE 4.
(A,B) Location and approach for an intra-articular injection of the knee.

Anserine Bursa

The pes anserine bursa is located proximal to the insertion site for the semitendinosus, gracilis, and sartorius tendons onto the proximal medial tibia. With the patient seated and the knee flexed 90°, the needle is inserted to the tibial periosteum at the point of greatest tenderness and is withdrawn slightly before injection.

Ankle

Intra-articular Space

Intra-articular injection of the ankle is rarely indicated or attempted. Aspiration of this joint may provide important diagnostic information. The ankle joint is entered just medial to the tibialis anterior tendon. The needle should be held parallel to the superior surface of the talus and should not be directed distally toward the foot.

Foot

Plantar Fascia

In a review of treatment options for plantar fasciitis, Buchbinder [40] found limited evidence that corticosteroid injection provides short-term benefit. Despite the lack of evidence, corticosteroid injection is considered an initial treatment option for plantar fasciitis (grade of recommendation: D) [40]. At the site of origin of the plantar fascia from the calcaneus, the area of greatest tenderness is determined. A plantar or medial approach is used, although a medial approach may assist in preserving the tissue integrity of the sole. The needle is directed toward the insertion of the plantar fascia into the calcaneus.

Key Points

- Aspiration of synovial fluid and injection of joints, bursae, tendon sheaths, and soft tissues are diagnostic and therapeutic skills used by physicians practicing in the outpatient setting.
- Aspiration of synovial fluid is indicated to further evaluate a spontaneous, unexplained joint effusion with or without associated trauma if the diagnosis is uncertain.
- Injection of joints and soft tissues is used for both diagnosis and treatment of numerous musculoskeletal diagnoses.
- Intra- and peri-articular steroid injections have been found to be a safe procedure with a very low complication rate if performed while taking adequate precautions, including post-injection infection rats of 1:16,000 to 1-2:150,000 have been cited.
- The medical benefits of intra-articular and soft tissue injection are inconsistent and appear to be affected by numerous variables, including diagnosis, site of injection, medications used, and additional incorporated therapies.
- Currently, the literature consistently supports local injection for lateral epicondylitis and carpal tunnel syndrome and intra-articular injection of the knee for underlying osteoarthritis and bursitis.

References

[1] Hollander J. Intra-articular hydrocortisone in arthritis and allied conditions. J Bone Joint Surg 1953;35A:983–90.
[2] Carek PJ, King DE, Abercrombie S. does community or university-based residency sponsorship affect practice profiles? Fam Med 2002;34:592–7.

[3] Godwin M, Dawes M. Intra-articular steroid injections for painful knees. Can Fam Physician 2004;50:241–8.

[4] Arroll B, Goodyear-Smith F. Corticosteroid injections for osteoarthritis of the knee: meta-analysis. BMJ 2004;328:869.

[5] Anderson B, Kaye S. Treatment of flexor tenosynovitis of the hand ('trigger finger') with corticosteroids: a prospective study of the response to local injection. Arch Intern Med 1991;151:153–6.

[6] Buchbinder R, Green S, Youd JM. Corticosteroid injections for shoulder pain. Cochrane Database Syst Rev 2003;1:CD004016.

[7] Kolba KS. The approach to the acute joint and synovial fluid examination. Prim Care 1984;11:211–8.

[8] Shmerling RH. Synovial fluid analysis: a critical appraisal. Rheum Dis Clin North Am 1994;20:503–12.

[9] Klippel JH, Weyand CM, Crofford LH, et al, editors. Primer on the rheumatic diseases. 12th edition. Atlanta (GA): Arthritis Foundation; 2001.

[10] Pfenniger JL. Injections of joints and soft tissue: part I. General guidelines. Am Fam Physician 1991;44:1196–202.

[11] Cardone DA, Tallia AF. Joint and soft tissue injection. Am Fam Physician 2002;66: 283–8.

[12] Pfenniger JL. Injections of joints and soft tissue: Part II. General guidelines. Am Fam Physician 1991;44:1690–701.

[13] Schaffer TC. Joint and soft-tissue arthocentesis. Prim Care 1993;20:757–70.

[14] Kerlan RK, Glousman RE. Injections and techniques in athletic medicine. Clin Sports Med 1989;8:541–60.

[15] Kelly MA, Kurzweil PR, Moskowitz RW. Intra-articular hyalurons in knee osteoarthritis: rationale and practical considerations. Am J Orthopedics 2004;33(Suppl): 15–22.

[16] Aggarwal A, Sempowski IP. Hyaluronic acid injections for knee osteoarthritis: systemic review of the literature. Can Fam Physician 2004;50:249–56.

[17] Wang CT, Lin J, Chang CJ, et al. Therapeutic effects of hyaluronic acid on osteoarthritis of the knee. J Bone Joint Surg 2004;86A:538–45.

[18] Leopold SS, Redd BB, Warme WJ, et al. Corticosteroid compared with hyaluronic acid injections for the treatment of osteoarthritis of the knee. J Bone Joint Surg 2003;85A: 1197–203.

[19] Donnelly AJ, Shafer AL. Perioperative care. In: Young LY, Koda-Kimble MA, editors. Applied therapeutics: the clinical use of drugs. Vancouver: Applied Therapeutics; 1995. p. 1–24.

[20] Owens DS. Aspiration and injection of joints and soft tissue. In: Ruddy S, Harris ED, Sledge CB, editors. Kelley's textbook of rheumatology. 6th edition. Philadephia: W.B. Saunders; 2001. p. 583–603.

[21] Zuckerman JD, Meslin RJ, Rothberg M. Injections for joint and soft tissue disorders: when and how to use them. Geriatrics 1990;45:45–52, 55.

[22] Gray RG, Gottlieb NL. Intra-articular corticosteroids: an updated assessment. Clin Orthop 1983;177:235–63.

[23] Kumar N, Newman RJ. Complications of intra- and peri-articular steroid injections. Br J Gen Pract 1999;49:465–6.

[24] Hollander JL. Arthrocentesis and instrasynovial therapy. In: McCarty DJ, editor. Arthritis and allied conditions. 9th edition. Philadelphia: Lea & Febiger; 1979. p. 402–14.

[25] Stefanich RJ. Intraarticular corticosteroids in treatment of osteoarthritis. Orthop Rev 1986;15:65–71.

[26] Pal B, Morris J. Perceived risks of joint infection following intra-articular corticosteroid injections: a survey of rheumatologists. Clin Rheum 1999;18:264–5.

[27] Charalambous CP, Tryfonidis M, Sadiq S, et al. Septic arthritis following intra-articular steroid injection of the knee: a survey of current practice regarding antiseptic technique used during intra-articular steroid injection of the knee. Clin Rheum 2003;22:386–90.

[28] Black DM, Filak AT. Hyperglycemia with non-insulin-dependent diabetes following intraarticular steroid injection. J Fam Pract 1989;28:462–3.

[29] Bostron P, Calver R. Subcutaneous atrophy following methylprednisolone injection in Osgood-Schlatter epiphysitis. J Bone Joint Surg 1979;61A:627–8.

[30] van der Heijden GJ, van der Windt DA, Kleijnen J, et al. Steroid injections for shoulder disorders: a systematic review of randomized clinical trials. Br J Gen Pract 1996;46: 309–16.

[31] Assendelft WJ, Hay EM, Adshead R, et al. Corticosteroid injections for lateral epicondylitis: a systematic overview. Br J Gen Pract 1996;46:209–16.

[32] Smidt N, van der Windt DA, Assendelft WJ, et al. Corticosteroid injections, physiotherapy, or a wait-and-see policy for lateral epicondylitis: a randomised controlled trial. Lancet 2002;359:657–62.

[33] Bowen RE, Dorey FJ, Shapiro MS. Efficacy of nonoperative treatment for lateral epicondylitis. Am J Ortho 2001;30:642–6.

[34] Newport ML, Lane LB, Stuchin SA. Treatment of trigger finger by steroid injection J Hand Surg 1990;15:748–50.

[35] Murphy D, Failla JM, Koniuch MP. Steroid versus placebo injection for trigger finger J Hand Surg 1995;20:628–31.

[36] Lane LB, Boretz RS, Stuchin SA. Treatment of de Quervain's disease: role of conservative management. J Hand Sur (Br) 2001;26:258–60.

[37] Marshall S, Tardiff G, Ashworth N. Local corticosteroid injection for carpal tunnel syndrome. Cochrane Database Syst Rev 2002;4, CD001554.

[38] Ege Rasmussen KJ, Fano N. Trochanteric bursitis: treatment by corticosteroid injection. Scand J Rheum 1985;14:417–20.

[39] Raynauld J, Buckland-Wright C, Ward R, et al. Safety and efficacy of long-term intraarticular steroid injections in osteoarthritis of the knee. Arth Rheum 2003;48:370–7.

[40] Buchbinder R. Plantar fasciitis. N Engl J Med 2004;350:2159–66.

Address reprint requests to

Peter J. Carek, MD, MS
Department of Family Medicine
Medical University of South Carolina
9298 Medical Plaza Drive, Charleston, SC 29406

e-mail: carekpj@musc.edu

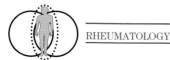

Note: Page numbers of article titles are in **boldface** type.